# STYLE CLINIC

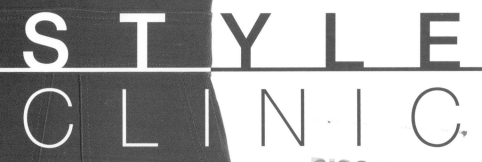

# STYLE
# CLINIC

HOW TO LOOK
FABULOUS ALL THE TIME,
AT ANY AGE,
FOR ANY OCCASION

PAULA REED

**COLLINS** LIVING
*An Imprint of HarperCollins Publishers*

FIRST EDITION

*Designed by Agnieszka Stachowicz*

Library of Congress Cataloging-in-Publication Data is available upon request.

ISBN 978-0-06-079354-8

09  10  11  12  13   OV/RRD   10 9 8 7 6 5 4 3 2 1

# CONTENTS

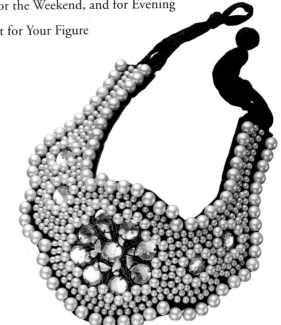

# INTRODUCTION

I'VE BEEN A FASHION EDITOR for twenty years now. I've worked in London and New York, zigzagged the world over at the merest hint of a hot trend, used planes like buses in pursuit of the latest style icons, and spent more hours than I care to count waiting for the unveiling of the coolest fashion happening. I was there for John Galliano's first show and shed a tear at Yves Saint Laurent's last. And, after years of front-row fashion show action and privileged access, I can tell you, ladies, that in a world of "it" bags, must-haves, and seasonal waiting lists, one thing I know for sure is true: Fashion is a fleeting pleasure. Style is like an enduring affair with someone who loves you back.

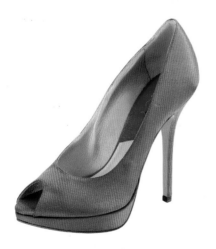

In all the red-carpet, backstage, and front-row comings and goings in all that time, the women who made a splash in their seasonal big-ticket items blend into a blur of fashion blah. The stylish standouts are memorable still: the sixty-year-old Frenchwoman in tuxedo suit and heels making the rest of us in puffy dresses feel overdressed at a party in Paris; somebody's assistant looking so cool in jeans and her grandmother's jewelry when the rest of us were having our gothic Japanese moment; the coltish gatecrasher bouncing into one of those trophy store openings on Madison in ballerina shoes and bright orange Birkin bag when power suits and heels were the uniform *du jour*.

Real style, the kind that stops you in your tracks, is a thing some baby girls are just blessed with. It's in their DNA. Like flawless skin or a high-speed metabolism, they can take for granted what the rest of us have to work at. The good news, for those of us who have to work at it, is that style is an achievable goal. And before we go any further, let's get one major misconception straight: You don't need a lottery win to have it. In fact, a big budget often leads only to that tragic codependency that makes fashion conglomerates Fortune 500 companies and turns otherwise fabulous females into label victims.

Diana Vreeland, legendary editor of *Harper's Bazaar* and American *Vogue*, once said "Elegance is refusal." In simple terms, success is about is knowing what works for you and what would look better on someone else (maybe someone with another body, or just another life). Unless you can learn this, fashion will always fail you. And, no matter how many clothes you have, your wardrobe will have the last laugh in a fashion crisis. On the other hand, with a little basic skill, deftly applied, you can have the confidence that comes with knowing that what you put on in the morning looks great and, regardless of what your day might bring, need never be given another moment's thought.

This book is about helping you to get to the point where looking great is easy. It will offer tips and guidelines to help you find your way through the acres of choice. It'll reacquaint you with some simple fashion rules that somehow are forgotten in the rush to bag a big new trend. Having your own rule book is what stands between you and another fashion mistake. Remember: True fashion fabulousness lies in your own personal style.

This is not a textbook. You don't become perfectly dressed when you get to the last page. A few shopping lists and bullet points will give you ideas where to start. But don't lose heart. No one is born with an instinct about how to dress for every occasion. Even for the innately stylish, this is a skill that evolves over time, a confidence that comes from a constant process of trial and error. Throughout that process, this book will be your guide: a friendly insider who won't freak you out by speaking fashion gobbledygook. No one is going to insist you shoulder up to Kate Moss on the style grid. But every woman owes herself the simple pleasure of dressing well. Surrendering to frumpery is not an option.

So, if your wardrobe is a throwback to another time in your life (pre-baby, weight loss/gain, new job, relationship), or it's a muddle of old favorites, or you find yourself saying it's worked so far, why change it, step up for an overhaul. Beyond fashion there is a style that will do your uniqueness justice.

"STYLE IS VERY

FROM

ONCE YOU FIND

THAT WORKS,

**DIFFERENT**

FASHION.

SOMETHING

**KEEP IT."**

# 1

## WARDROBE

## R E H A B

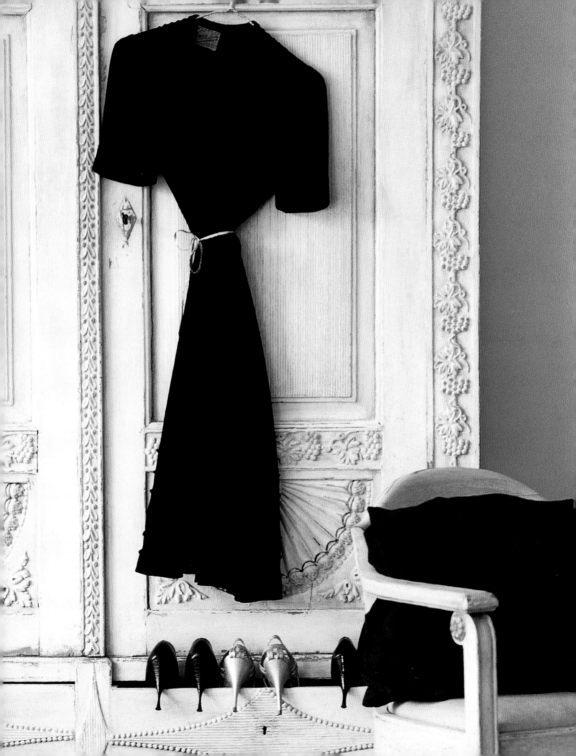

**I LOVE AMERICA,** AND I LOVE AMERICAN WOMEN.
**BUT THERE IS ONE THING**
THAT DEEPLY SHOCKS ME—**AMERICAN CLOSETS.**
I CANNOT BELIEVE ONE CAN DRESS WELL
**WHEN YOU HAVE SO MUCH.**

Andrée Putman, legendary French interior designer

LET ME GUESS. If you've come this far, chances are your closet is too full of stuff you never wear: all-time favorites, one-season wonders, and bargains you always thought you could slim down and fit into. Filleting out fashion mistakes is tough. But it is time for action if:

- What's in your wardrobe has become a mystery to you. You have no idea what you own because everything is stuffed in together.

- At the end of a season your wardrobe is full of unworn clothes and things that don't work with more than one outfit.

- Getting dressed has become a chore and looking good is a grind. What stands between you and looking fabulous is some tough decisions. But the results are so worth it. "Effortless chic" is fashion's biggest lie. Great wardrobes don't just happen.

## WHAT TO KEEP AND WHAT TO DITCH

Let's be clear about one thing: Getting a great wardrobe is not about being spoiled or self-obsessed. Knowing what you have and how it works for you saves you time and will

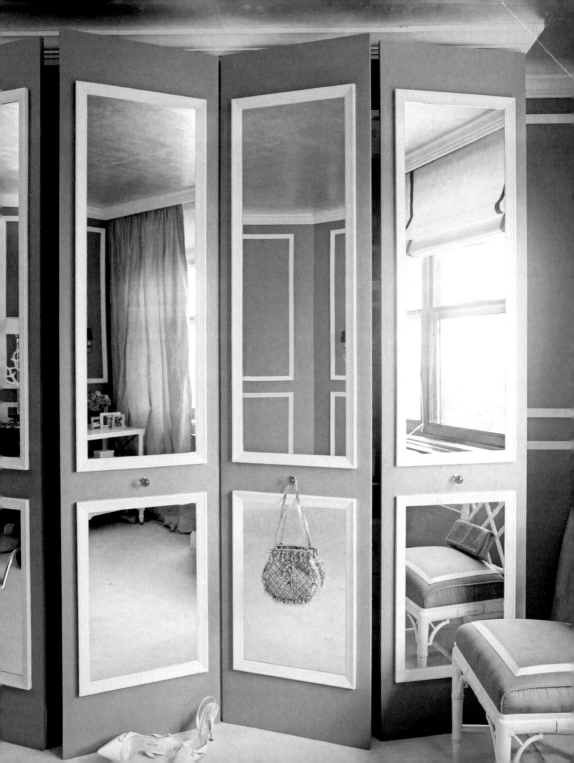

give you peace of mind when you need to know you look good. You can look great, every day, with minimal fuss.

You may never be satisfied that the job is done. This doesn't matter. It may never be done. But knowing what you need makes you a better shopper, less likely to be tempted by impulse buys. And being able to see just what you have can inspire outfits you didn't even know you had. Old favorites become new looks when you spot combinations you never considered.

If, throughout this process, you can be as honest and ruthless as possible (or, failing that, find a friend who will be), you'll quickly begin to find out what works and what doesn't. The things that work are the elements of your personal style, the basis of your own personal fashion rule book. With time and confidence, your rules may be bent, but never, ever broken.

If the job seems enormous, don't worry. Getting started is the hardest part.

## KNOW YOUR STYLE

### PLAN

You can't do this in an hour, so make sure you set aside enough time. A day should be enough to reorganize shelving and hanging space, but if there is any DIY involved (repainting, shelf hanging), you'll need two days. Have all the things you need at hand: a full-length mirror, garbage bags, hangers (see page 24 for the essential wardrobe kit).

### PURGE

Empty your wardrobe completely. Immediately cut your task in half by setting aside out-of-season clothes. This is only a temporary measure, but it feels so good to get fast results. That set-aside stuff will eventually need to be sorted, but at least you can tackle it later.

### SORT

Try everything on. If it no longer fits (your look, your shape, your taste), get rid of it. Make five separate piles of clothes for the

SOMEONE ONCE SAID, **"GENIUS IS THE CAPACITY FOR TAKING INFINITE PAINS."** THEREFORE, WHEN DRESSING, BE ABSORBED COMPLETELY AND UTTERLY IN YOURSELF, **LETTING NO DETAIL ESCAPE YOU.** HOWEVER, ONCE DRESSED, **BE INTERESTED ONLY IN THOSE ABOUT YOU.**

Diana Vreeland

dry cleaner, the tailor, the charity shop, the trash, and eveningwear. You may end up with an "iffy" pile, but don't let it get too big. The trash and charity piles should not be left lying around or they'll creep back into your wardrobe. Some charities and recycling companies will collect old clothes. Call them immediately.

Failing that, turn your trash into cash by having a yard sale or taking a stand at a flea market. Gently worn or collectible labels can go on eBay. Or, even better, plan a swap party: Your fashion mistake could easily be your girlfriend's dream dress. What remains can, collectively, be dispatched to the charity shop.

DITCH

- All clothes that have shiny, worn patches on the seat or the knees.
- All clothes that show the shape of your butt or knees when you are not in them.
- All clothes that are beyond the help of the best tailor you can find. The telephone numbers of experts like these are often one of a stylish woman's best-kept secrets. Failing that, good stores generally have a direct line to the best alterations people. Be brazen. If you don't ask, you don't get.
- All clothes that are too small or too large.
- Anything that's not clothing (wrapping paper, photos, and books belong somewhere else).

If you're still having trouble working out what to ditch, put it in the iffy pile and apply the two-year rule: If you haven't worn something in that long, it has to go; there is no excuse. Once that's done, only the best of what you have remains in the cupboard.

## The Only Exceptions

- Eveningwear. It gets worn less and so, if it's stored correctly, stays in good condition for longer. And classic trends always come back.

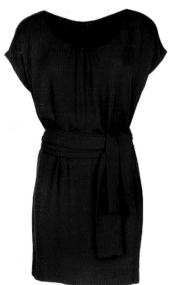

*Your Favorite Color*

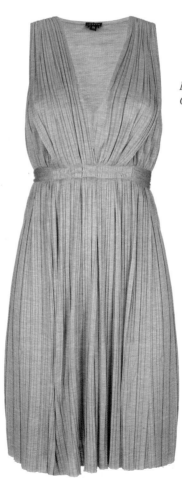

*Dateless
Day-to-Evening
Dress*

*Evening
Classic*

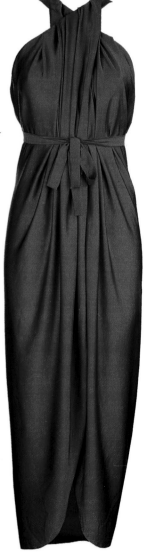

- Stuff you think is collectible (don't you envy your friends whose moms kept their Halstons?). By all means keep your favorite fashion moments for posterity, but that doesn't mean those harem pants should get another airing in your lifetime.

- Anything that has made it through all these filters because of its fantastic quality. Keep these in a box with all the other iffy items for annual reassessment.

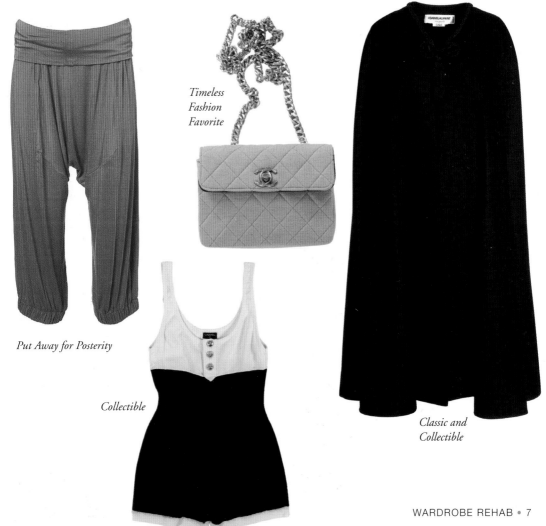

*Timeless Fashion Favorite*

*Put Away for Posterity*

*Collectible*

*Classic and Collectible*

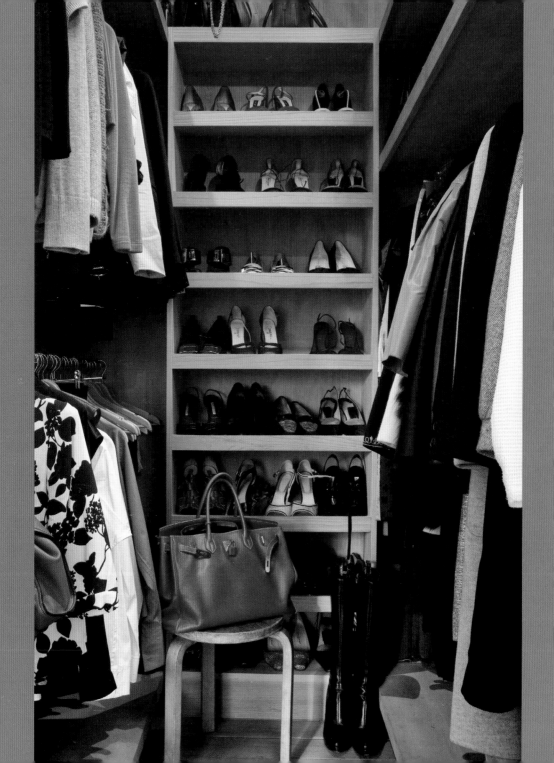

## YOUR NEW ORDER

When you put everything back in your
wardrobe, try to work out a way of arranging
things so you will know immediately where
to look for things. Here's my running order,
but feel free to adapt to whatever works
for you:

- Tops (shirts, shells, cardigans)
- Bottoms (pants, jeans, khakis, skirts)
- Tailored jackets (hanging with the
  skirts or pants they go with)
- Dresses (progressing from casual
  to evening)
- Eveningwear and coats (should have a
  little section of their own)

Don't forget: Put the out-of-season stuff
away. No one wears flannel in July. And
February is no time for a pretty peasant skirt.

## ALL DONE?
## KEEP UP THE GOOD WORK!

- Try to be organized about putting things
  back where they belong. That way you can
  avoid another long solitary confinement
  in the closet.

- Use spring and autumn to ritually
  reassess your wardrobe.

- Keep a notebook handy so you can jot
  down, at any time it occurs to you,
  what you need to make an outfit special
  or complete. You can add the contents to
  your holiday or birthday list.

- Clutter is the enemy. You can't have a
  vision if you can't see the stuff that will
  inspire you. At the end of each season,
  take stock.

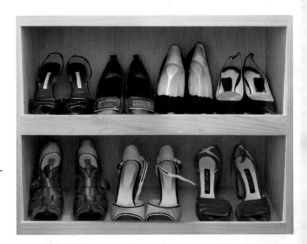

# 2

## WARDROBE

## B A S I C S

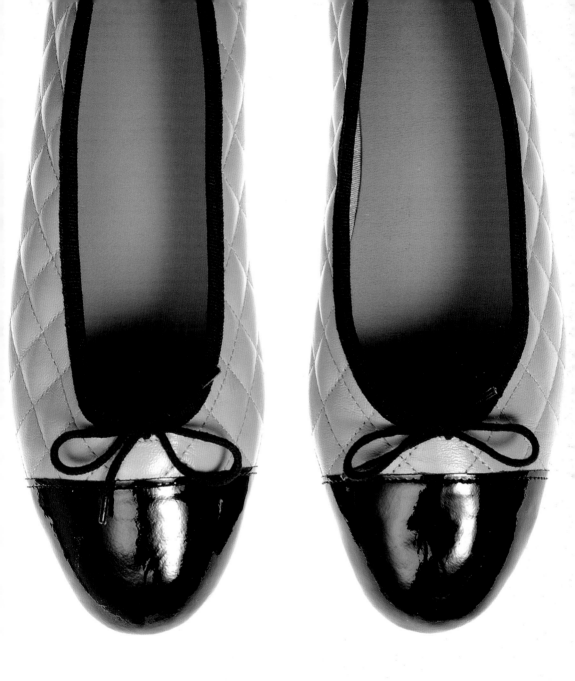

**ONE SHOULDN'T SPEND** ALL ONE'S TIME DRESSING. ALL ONE NEEDS ARE **TWO OR THREE SUITS,** AS LONG AS THEY, AND EVERYTHING TO GO WITH THEM, **ARE PERFECT.**

Coco Chanel

SO NOW YOU HAVE DONE your housekeeping. Bet you think you need loads of new stuff. But before you hit the stores, remember: You *can* have too many clothes. Better to have a few good things that are really you than roomfuls of stuff and still nothing to wear.

If you don't know where to start, try this. Whatever your lifestyle, every woman needs something to wear to

- A casual lunch with friends
- A job interview or business meeting
- A date
- A black-tie affair

## WHAT EVERY WARDROBE NEEDS

Here is a checklist of the bare essentials. It's not the last word. Think of it as a skeleton. How you flesh it out depends entirely on your own style. Go through it and your wardrobe and make notes about what's missing from your closet.

1. A sharp white shirt in a cut that best suits your figure
2. One very well made, lightweight cardigan in your favorite color
3. A jacket that works with your skirt (it will turn it into a suit)
4. Three pairs of trousers: denim, tailored for daywear, and smart (day-to-evening)

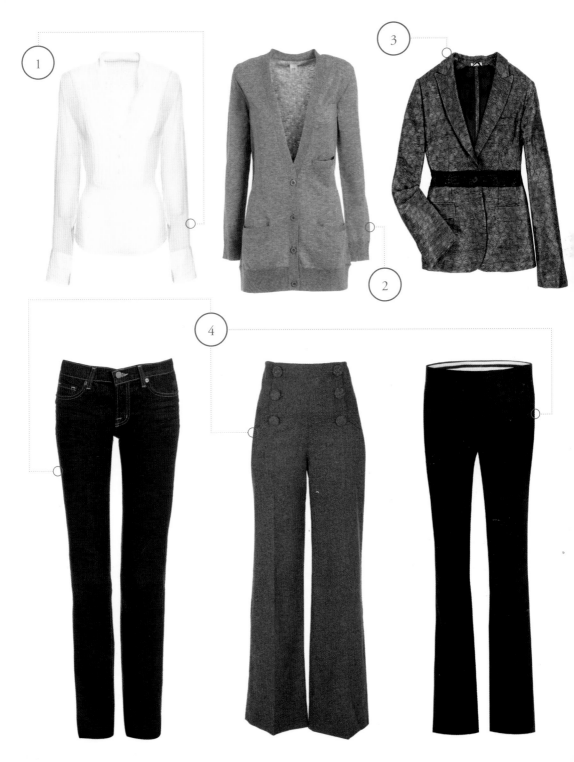

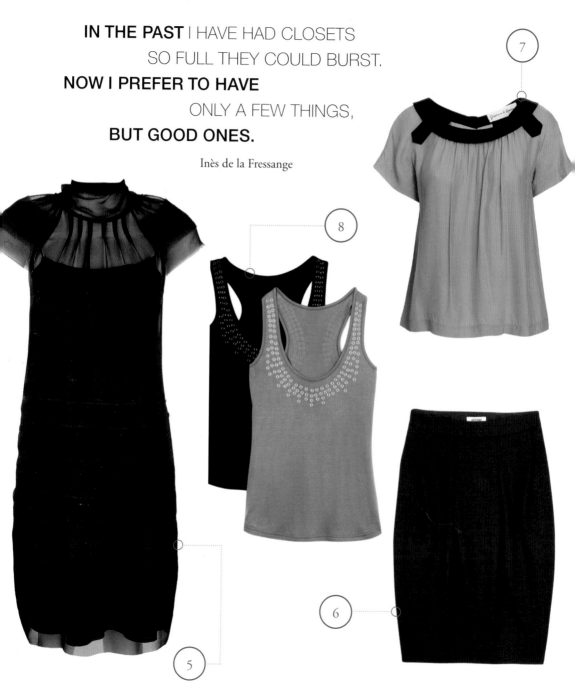

**IN THE PAST** I HAVE HAD CLOSETS
SO FULL THEY COULD BURST.
**NOW I PREFER TO HAVE**
ONLY A FEW THINGS,
**BUT GOOD ONES.**

Inès de la Fressange

5. One little black dress

6. A skirt that works for day, in a shape that suits your figure

7. A sleeveless or short-sleeved round-neck top (as a dressy alternative to the T-shirt)

8. A selection of simple T-shirts or tanks (black, white, and gray are the best basic range)

9. Three pairs of good shoes: boots, ballet flats or loafers, and a pair of evening shoes

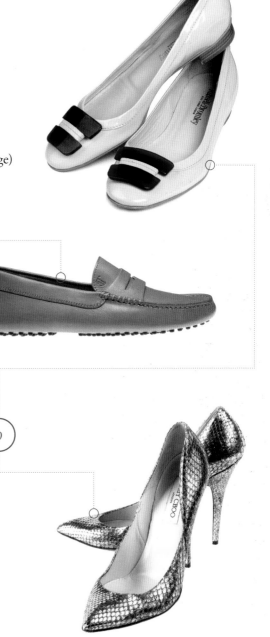

Okay, so you do also need other things (a great coat, knitwear, hanging-out-at-home-wear, eveningwear, and sneakers). And then, of course, some women already have their uniform. You might live in jeans, full stop. A uniform that works for you is a gift from the fashion gods. Stick with it. But be sure you eke out its full potential.

Another consideration: The fewer places you have to go, the smaller the wardrobe you need. But, even if you work from home or are momentarily out of work, you shouldn't assume you don't need a gorgeous pair of shoes and a simple tailored dress.

Armed with the list of essentials, topped up with your own requirements, go through your wardrobe again. Be ruthlessly honest about where the gaps are. This takes a will of iron. If you haven't got one, try role-playing. Sometimes, thinking of your stuff as if it were someone else's helps. Bear in mind that if something was trendy three years ago, chances are it's not at all cool today. No amount of money spent justifies keeping a mistake. Just console yourself that you won't make the same mistake again as you consign it to the reject bin.

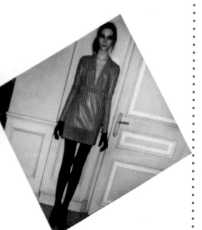

## UNIVERSAL STYLE TRUTH

A friend with a hard heart and great taste will be an ally when weeding out your wardrobe. Get her to take pictures of you in the outfits you aren't sure about. If you dither, the camera will be tougher than both of you.

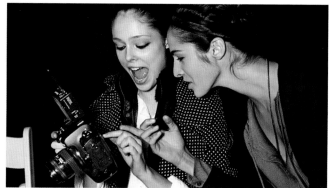

## HOW TO TAKE ON A TREND

If you think you already have something for every category above, go back and look again. If you have an expensive pair of black trousers you have hardly ever worn, it probably means they are not the right pair for you. Take them out of your closet.

Don't kid yourself that classic items never change. They evolve (slowly), but enough to leave you out if you don't keep reviewing your wardrobe. Fashion items come and go, so it's best to buy inexpensive versions of passing trends and dispense with them at the end of a season. Your classics, on the other hand, are likely to cost serious cash. They are the heart of your style. So don't let your fashion house crumble for want of a solid foundation. Subtle adjustments will make the difference between bringing your basics up-to-date and looking like you are someone's mother.

Be ruthlessly honest. You can be sure that one day your coolest dress will look too short or long. Your favorite jacket will suddenly look dowdy. The classic black skirt that cost a fortune and has worked so well for . . . ummm . . . several seasons, now looks too full. Trust your instinct on this one. If, one day, you suspect that cardigan would look better with a slimmer skirt or a leaner trouser, and your jeans could look chic with a slimmer or baggier white shirt, you're probably right.

The February and August issues of fashion magazines start to feature the new season's trends. A passing glance will give you pointers on where fashion is headed.

## BEWARE THE FRUMP FACTOR

It can kill a great look faster than Britney Spears. And it can creep up on anybody. Here's where you're most likely to find it:

- Shoulder pads (are they neat and narrow or wide right now?)
- Waistbands (this season, are they on the waist, low-slung, cinched?)
- Trouser legs (are current trends wide, narrow, straight, flared, boot-cut?)
- Heels (are they chunky, spiky, high, or low?)

- Hem lengths (what works now: long or short?)

A word to the wise: In fifty years of seasonally changing fashion, a skirt that just covers the wrinkly part of the knee never made a fool of anyone over twenty-five.

## REASONS TO RENEW

Keep the following things looking box fresh. Unless you are loaded, there is no need to buy designer versions of any of these. It's better to buy cheaply and replace as soon as they look less than perfect. That yellowing T-shirt doesn't fool anyone and, from the outside, no one can see the Jil Sander label.

- White shirts
- T-shirts
- Hosiery

## FASHION'S FAB FOUR: HOW TO GET MORE BANG FOR YOUR BASICS

## ALL A WOMAN NEEDS TO BE CHIC IS A RAINCOAT, TWO SUITS, A PAIR OF TROUSERS, AND A CASHMERE SWEATER.

Hubert de Givenchy

Mr. Givenchy's basic list is still pretty good. Maybe a twenty-first-century tweak would acknowledge that separates could take you more places than suits, that tailored trousers have moved way up the scale of importance, and that a great dress solves the day-to-evening style conundrum for millions of time-poor women. However you organize your life, fashion's fab four are vital elements of your fashion foundation. Here's how to make them work for you.

## THE WHITE SHIRT

There are those who swear that the only way to get close to perfection here is to go for budget-busting designer quality. Others think that, to look sharp, you need to go for the best cut among the most affordable ranges

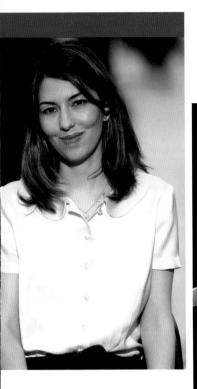

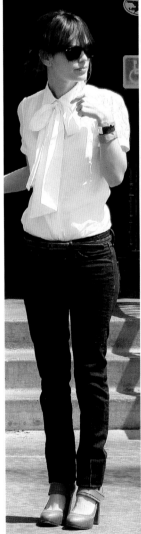

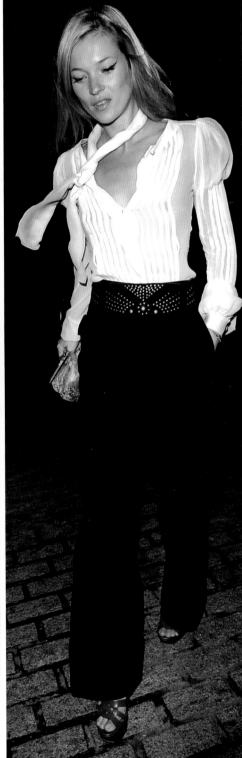

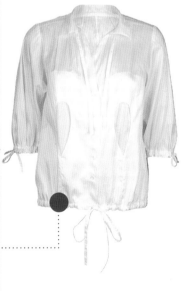

so you can replace this queen of the staples at the first sign of shabbiness. I've tried both ways. I think grimy urban living makes the disposable white shirt the only option.

How to Wear It

- Buy one that is classically cut, but with a slight edge. It could be a masculine detail such as a double cuff (in which case, try leaving them open and poking out at the cuff of a sweater or wearing cufflinks).

- Try a textured fabric such as cotton piqué, which always looks crisp. Avoid shiny synthetics. They look tacky.

- Go for a slim-cut over baggy, if you have the choice. A slight stretch will mean you feel comfortable (the ease you project when you are comfortable is one of the greatest but unsung secrets of chic).

- Choose a slightly drapey fabric and the effect is immediately sexy. Leave the top two buttons undone, but don't go for cleavage overkill.

- Tuck your shirt into skirts, but try leaving it out over slim pants (a figure-skimming cut is best for this).

- A cool white shirt and rugged jeans are a classic combination. A chunky belt is the perfect way to bridge the gap from cool whiteness to hot denim.

- Wear it with masculine pants and high-heeled shoes. Or try the same combination with mannish shoes, but finish it off with very feminine earrings. The combination of masculine restraint with one feminine element is red-hot.

- Wear it with a long, slim black skirt and killer jewelry for a stunningly simple evening option. Use your jewelry judiciously. The simplicity is a perfect backdrop for a big brooch (try it on the waistband of your skirt), a major cocktail ring, or a head-turning collar of pearls or stones. Two out of these three pieces is probably enough.

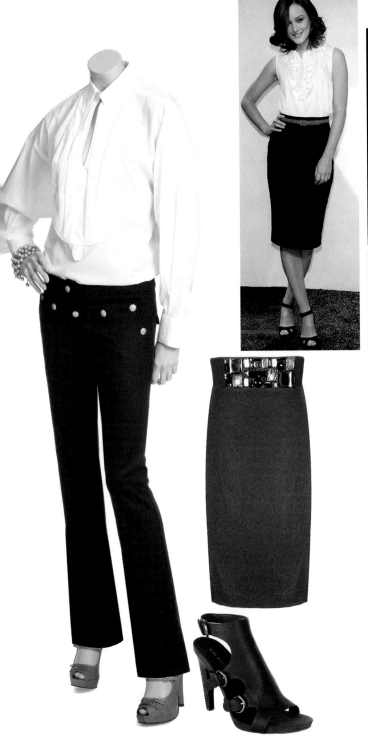

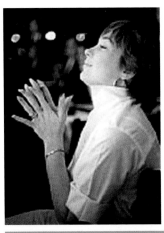

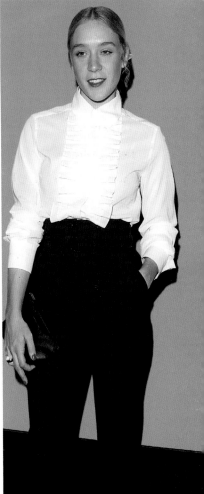

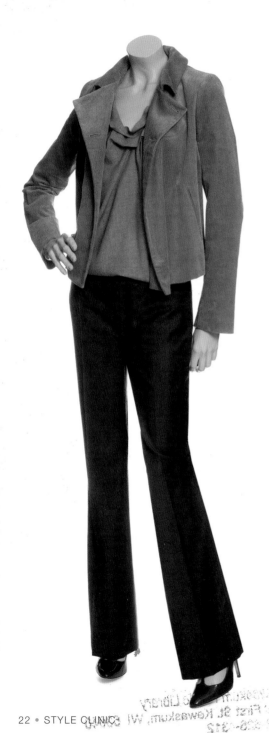

## THE JACKET

A jacket is the starting point for so many great looks. Whether you add tailored pants, a skirt, jeans or short shorts, whether you go funky or formal—these things are all about your personal style and way of life. No matter who you are, the jacket is king. Go for a simple cut in a fabric and color that will not easily date and will make the transition from season to season: Lightweight wool gabardine is fluid and elegant. Rayon (viscose) crepe is a magic silhouette smoother. Neat-shouldered, single-breasted jackets are kindest to most figures. Jackets with cardigan ease are the foundation on which Chanel based a fashion empire and are perfect for those allergic to formal tailoring. A jacket that covers most of your bottom suits most bodies best (Buster Keaton is a bad role model). And, while making sure you have the basics covered, avoid details like big lapels or buttons that think they are jewelry: They limit the life of your jacket.

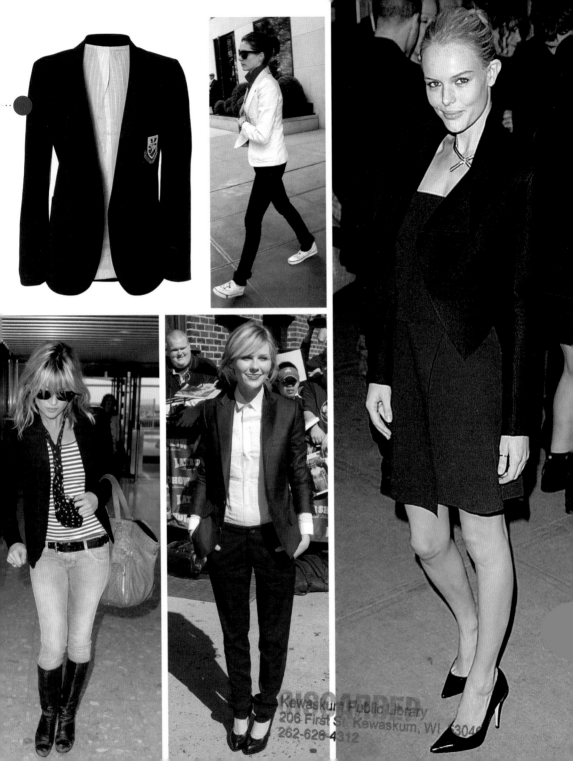

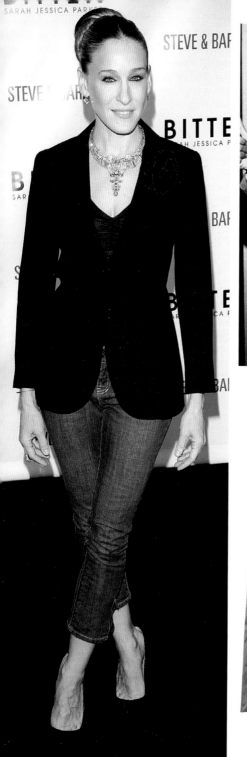
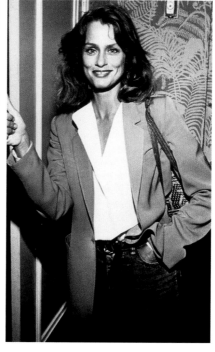
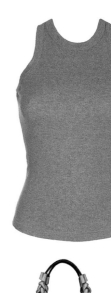
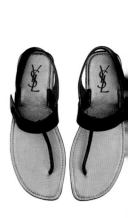
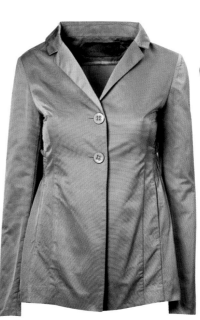

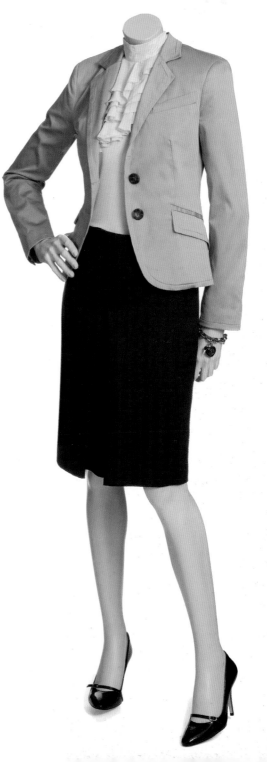

How to Wear It

- Wearing a single-breasted suit with a super-feminine underlayer, such as a lace camisole or chiffon slip, is not the latest fashion trick but always looks great.

- Try keeping your jacket buttoned up with a shirt and tie. Lighten the masculine overload with one (and I mean one) piece of feminine jewelry.

- Try a plain-cut, silky blouse with a string of pearls.

- Try your jacket with pants and a tailored vest or plain white T-shirt. High-heeled shoes with all this understated masculinity would be the head-turning detail here.

- Wear it over a simple shift dress as an alternative to your skirt or pantsuit.

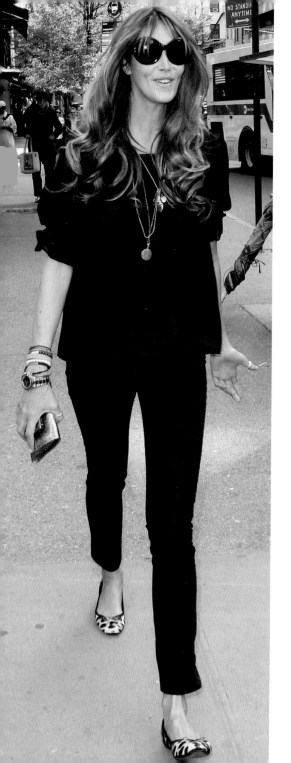

## YOUR PERFECT PANTS

Fashion trends come and go, but the flat-front, boot-leg trouser will always be the most adaptable shape in any wardrobe. They don't have to be tailored. Jeans and khakis count here, too.

**How to Wear Them**

- Avoid a tight fit at all costs: The squeezing adds pounds. Buy them figure-skimming, even if it means going up a size from what you normally wear. The effect is instantly slimming.

- A simple cut in a classic material is great. But the same shape in velvet, suede, or brocade becomes a style statement. Just don't let your top half or shoes compete for attention. A neat little sweater or sleeveless top will do.

- Try some alternative cocktail impact by dressing up your khakis or jeans with a billowing top and a piece of statement jewelry.

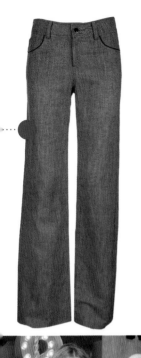

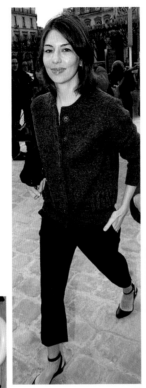

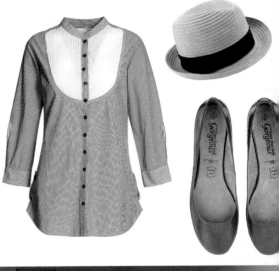

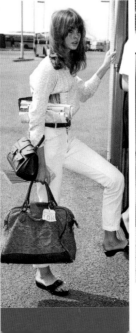

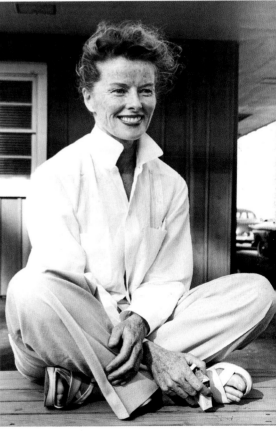

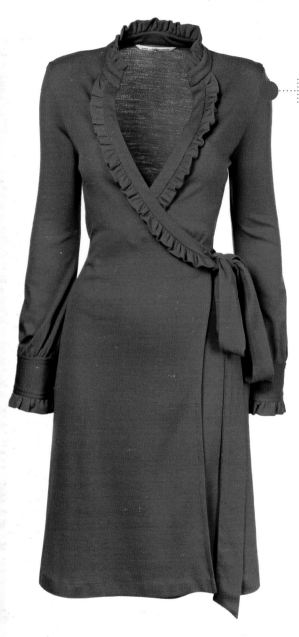

## THE DRESS

My desert island packing list will always feature a dress before a skirt. You put it on; you're done. No mucking around with what goes with it. As great as it is, the shift is not the last word in dresses. If you buy one great dress, make it as feminine as you dare. Even if your world is all about showing hard edges, a little softness can have a serious impact.

### How to Wear It

- If you have a favorite color that looks great on you, here is where you can go for it in a solid block.

- Go for a figure-skimming, not -hugging, line and a fabric that is fluid but not too fluttery. The flimsier the fabric, the more revealing it is. Chiffon is fabulous, but it needs a lining that effectively smoothes out everything underneath. Wool crepe, silk, rayon, and viscose with a touch of Lycra will all make you feel like a

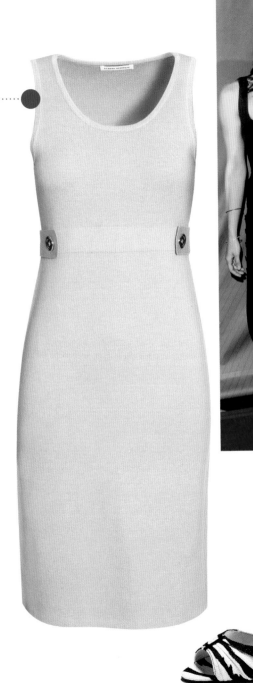

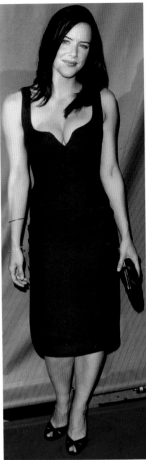

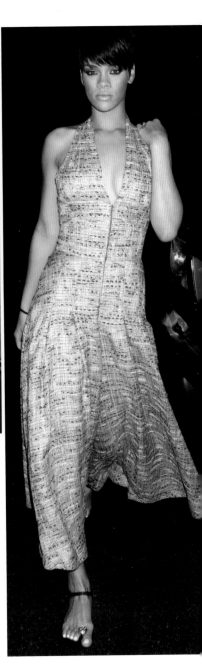

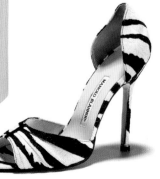

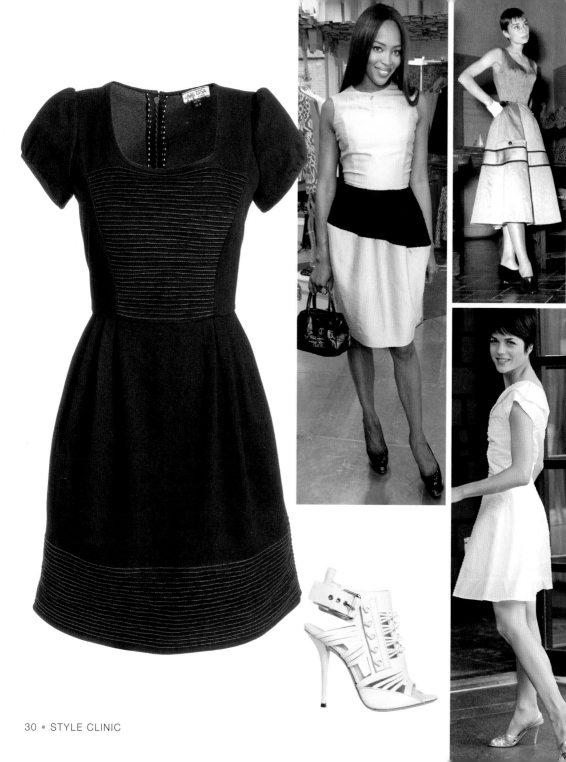

# FASHION MUST BE
## AN INTOXICATING RELEASE
### FROM **THE BANALITY**
## OF THE WORLD.

Diana Vreeland

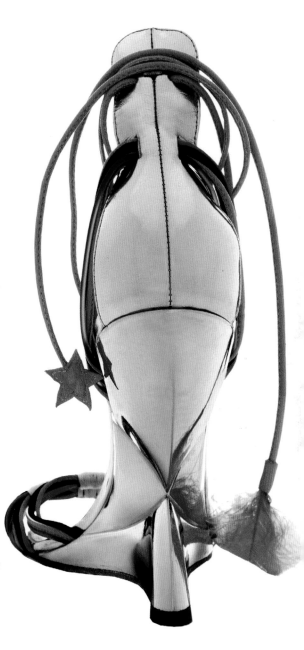

goddess. But a great quality matte jersey will magically smooth over your body's imperfections like a silken coverlet over a lumpy mattress.

- Let the fabric create the lightness. Avoid overexposure with acres of naked skin. Slip dresses have limited appeal and usefulness.

**Never forget:** The secret weapon of every stylish woman is that one unexpected item that turns a good look into an amazing one. It could be gorgeous shoes, a quirky bag, a piece of signature jewelry, or a weakness for hats. It's that bit of fantasy that keeps your clothes from looking too much like a uniform.

# 3

**FASHION'S ALL-TIME FAVORITE WARDROBE**

F    I    X    E    R    S

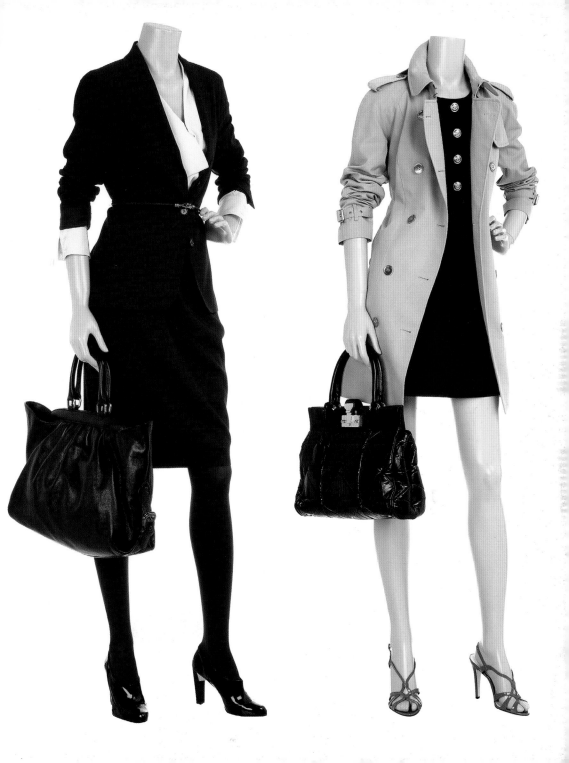

**FASHION IS LIKE THE ID.** IT MAKES YOU DESIRE THINGS **YOU SHOULDN'T.**

Bob Morris, travel writer and novelist

THE FICKLE FASHION FAN, whose wardrobe follows every catwalk U-turn, has always struck me as a girl with an identity crisis. For one woman with any kind of real life to segue without irony from prom queen to surfing cutie in one season demands a style-defying leap of logic.

Sooner or later, you have got to get over it. Life gets too full. You never have enough shoes. Or you simply begin to realize that trends are momentary thrills. You eventually know that, even if your reactions are lightning-sharp, the fashion gurus will speak, the tide of trends will turn, and last month's hot buy will look as appealing as cold pizza.

**SHE CAME INTO THE BAR OF THE RITZ** WEARING A KNEE-LENGTH TWEED SKIRT, A TWINSET, AND MOCCASINS**—AND IN A TIME WHEN** EVERYONE ELSE **WAS TARTED UP IN DIOR'S NEW LOOK,** SHE STOPPED TRAFFIC.

Bill Blass, describing C. Z. Guest in Paris in the 1950s

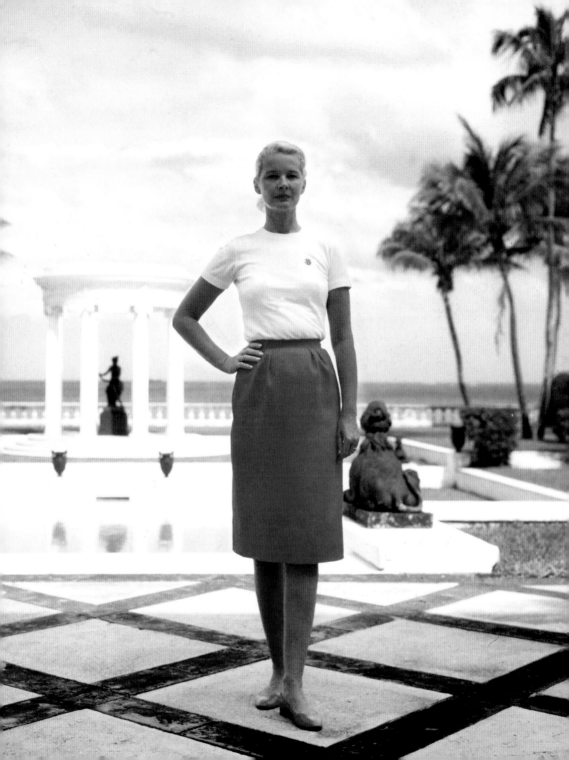

> I AM AGAINST FASHION **THAT DOESN'T LAST.**
> **I CANNOT ACCEPT** THAT
> YOU THROW YOUR CLOTHES AWAY
> **JUST BECAUSE IT IS SPRING.**
>
> Coco Chanel

Shop your style, not the hottest fashion trend. A forty-year-old working mother of three is unlikely to have been front of mind the day cropped tops were created. However, if you want to risk a crushed morale when next you find yourself cruelly exposed beside an abs-baring nineteen-year-old who clearly was, you have only yourself to blame. On the other hand, the diva dress that turns heads when you wear it would look ridiculous on her. Think about it. There's no mystery here.

None of this gives us an opt-out for seasonal renewal. Vitality is the key to great style. Having a clear sense of your fashion foundation and how to surf a trend will keep you and your wardrobe looking fresh, not frumpy. Only the queen of England, and a lady in waiting or two, can get away with picking a spot in fashion history and never changing a detail.

Here's how it works. If fashion's "fab four" (chapter 2) are your style foundation, what comes next is the structure. There are many options, but as you build your wardrobe and fine-tune your look, it's worth checking out the list below. They may not always be the hottest trend in town, but in thirty years, they have never been far from fashion's front line. Any time you feel your look has lost its luster, these things will always be right.

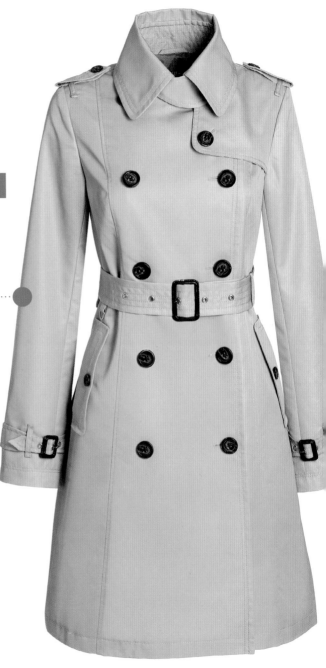

## THE CLASSICS

### THE TRENCH COAT

If the budget doesn't stretch to Burberry, then check out the details that make it so great before you go looking for the budget version—and don't compromise. Too much trench will swamp even tall women. Keep the shape neat. Avoid shoulders that are too big, hems that come to mid-calf (an inch or two below the knee is enough), and lapels that are too wide. Flapping around like a big beige bird is not the point.

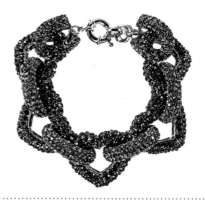

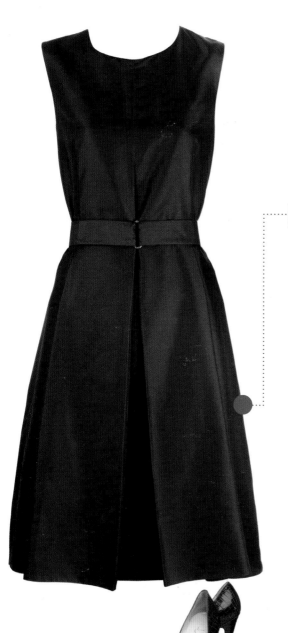

## THE LBD (LITTLE BLACK DRESS)

For its effortless transition from day through cocktails to eveningwear, my award for the most adaptable wardrobe item goes to the little black dress. Choose the shape that works best for you and it will never let you down. The tailored, V-neck shift is the best option if you are big-busted. Its structure is a great silhouette smoother. Boyish figures should go for round-necked, waisted shifts, which will add oomph. The lusciously curved, on the other hand, may want to try a shape with more swing in the skirt. It doesn't have to be full: Diane Von Fursten-berg's sexy jersey wrap drapes elegantly over those bootylicious curves. Whatever shape you decide is best, a rayon or wool crepe or good quality jersey with substantial weight will maximize its versatility.

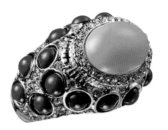

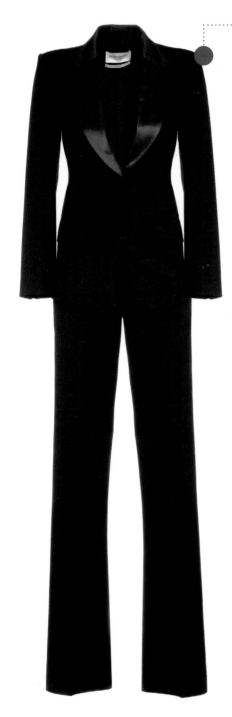

## THE TUXEDO SUIT

Launched by Yves Saint Laurent in the year
of the Rolling Stones's "19th Nervous Break-
down," this suit still smolders. (Jumping
Jack Flash is looking way more rumpled.) A
sharp-shouldered, single-breasted jacket with
notched lapels that can be worn with a pair
of straight-legged black pants is among the
most timeless, elegant, and useful things a
woman can have in her wardrobe.

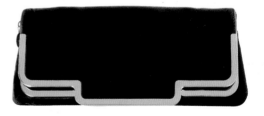

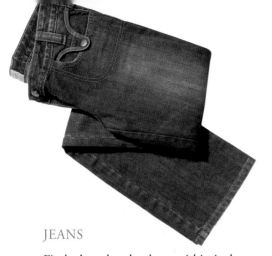

## JEANS

Find a brand and a shape within it that flatters your figure and stick with it. There is a hot new jeans shape every season. But if hip-slung boot-legged jeans make your legs look long and your butt look hot, then why on earth stray into shark territory of high waists and wide legs just because it's in fashion? By all means experiment, but your most successful ventures are likely to be within your favorite brand.

## CLASSIC KNITS

### 1.  The Twinset

Okay, so maybe this quaint twosome isn't the first thing that springs to mind for a twenty-first-century fashion list, but worn together or separately, there are several versatile options in this classic combo. Go for a fine

lamb's wool short-sleeved, round-necked sweater and a long-sleeved cardigan (if you're big-busted, create a streamlining V-neck by buttoning the bottom buttons only). Round necks that show the start of your collarbone look best. Either or both pieces look as good with jeans as with a straight knee-length skirt. The cardigan slung around the shoulders is the most charming chill chaser you'll ever see. And your cardigan buttoned over naked flesh (with maybe a hint of lacy lingerie showing) is irresistibly understated sex appeal.

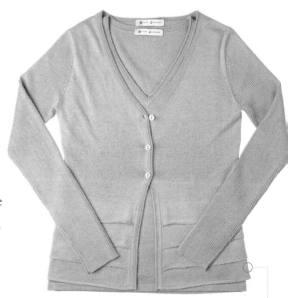

1

## 2. The Turtleneck Sweater

No single item can look as sharply dressed up one moment and laid back the next. It'll give your jeans a hint of Left Bank chic and bring some sleek luxury to your tailored trousers or slim skirt. Black is a timeless favorite, but a creamy white, rich camel, or rich chocolate brown are all great basics.

## 3. The Mannish V-Neck

Fashion heaven is my favorite pants and a sloppy mannish V-neck. That roomy shape hides a multitude of figure flaws, and the hint of skin is seriously sexy. Try it! The secret is to go for drape, not bulk, so choose sea island cotton or lightweight wool. Amp up the impact with killer heels and one piece of statement jewelry.

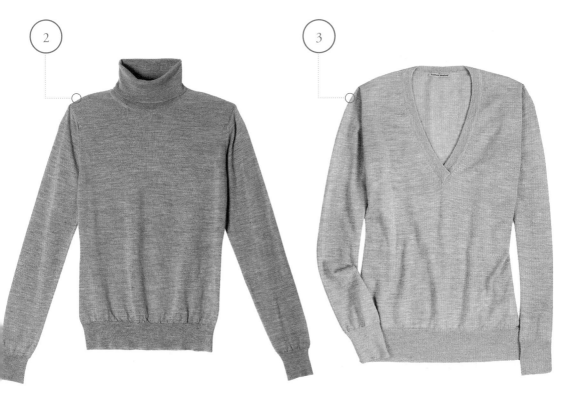

WHEN PUTTING A WARDROBE TOGETHER, IF YOUR BUDGET IS LIMITED, **THE MOST IMPORTANT THING IS** HAVING THE DISCIPLINE TO INVEST IN ONE OR TWO **BEAUTIFUL KEY PIECES** AND MIXING THESE WITH CLASSIC PIECES LIKE THE **CASHMERE SWEATER, THE GREAT JEAN, THE PERFECT CRISP WHITE SHIRT.** PLAN YOUR LONG-TERM WARDROBE. **ONLY BUY PIECES THAT YOU CAN'T LIVE WITHOUT;** DON'T BE TEMPTED **BY DISPOSABLE TRENDS.**

Roland Mouret

## ACCESSORIES

The big-ticket originals are budget breakers for all but billionaires. I live in eternal hope that one day my Birkin bag will come in. But hey, in the meantime, that doesn't stop anyone from checking out what makes these pieces great and applying what you learn to your next accessories purchase.

1. **The Hermès Kelly or Birkin Bag**

Great proportion, perfect size, mouthwatering colors. These are not just handbags, they're heirlooms. If the genuine article remains a remote possibility, find the closest approximation from among the thousands of great designs they have inspired.

2. **The Chanel Quilted Bag**

This one is never far from fashion-favorite status. The 2.55 is one of the great bags of all time.

3. **The Vuitton Sac Plat**

The perfect carryall. It can gobble up paperwork and still stand up and hold its open shape. A great working bag, this one is also a good, casual alternative to a handbag when you're wearing jeans.

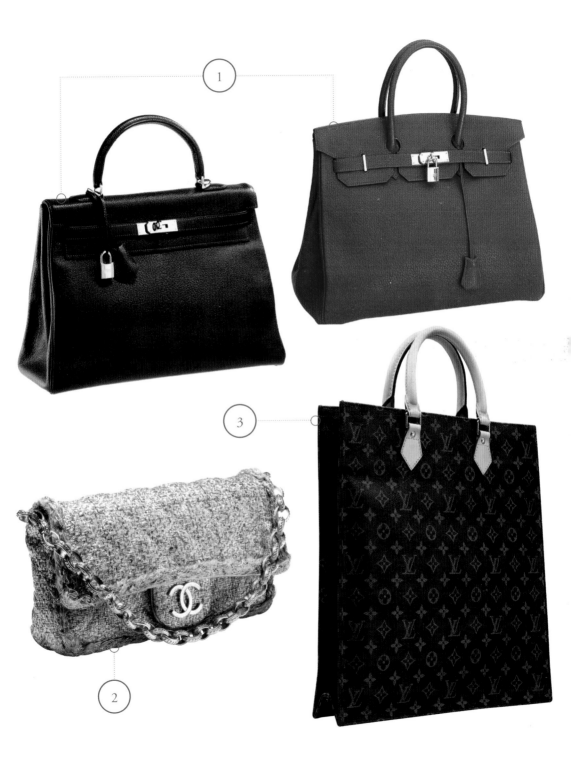

4. Bottega Veneta Cabat

Is it a purse, is it a tote? Who really cares? It's the most luxurious bag ever.

5. The L.L.Bean Canvas Tote

A preppy classic that has style credentials beyond the boating set.

6. Hermès H Belt

With jeans, over a sweater, nipping the waist through a tailored dress: It's perfect. Simple, elegant, and beautifully made. What more do you need?

7. Military Buckle Belt

As old as Elvis but still giving great hip action. Living proof that style icons look good dressed up or down. This one will do jeans, skirts, shift dresses, or tailored pants with equal ease. It's even been spotted on eveningwear, giving a simple dress some minimalist edge.

8. Converse Sneakers

The original and the best (and still under $50).

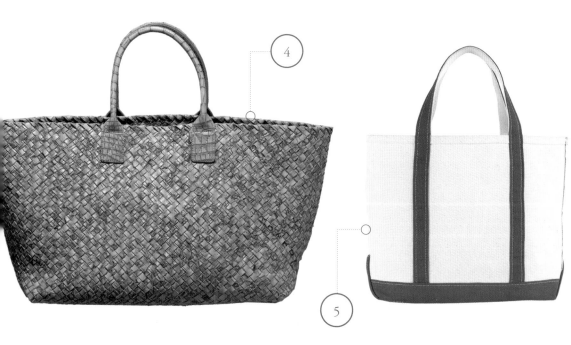

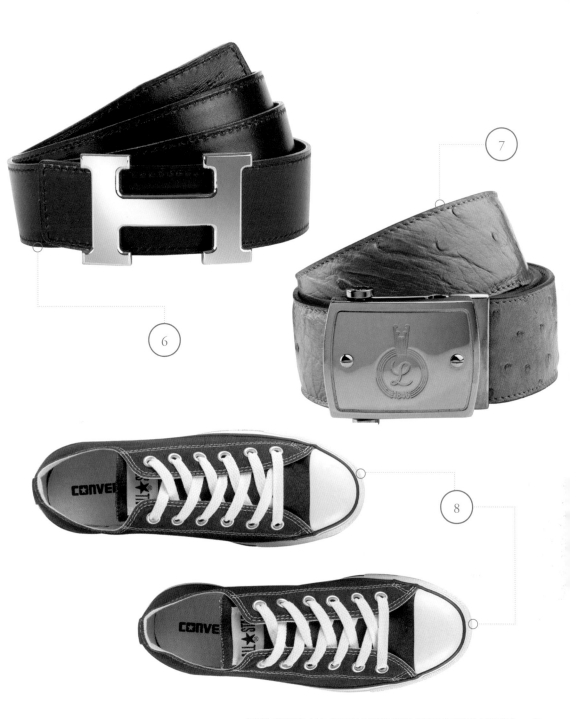

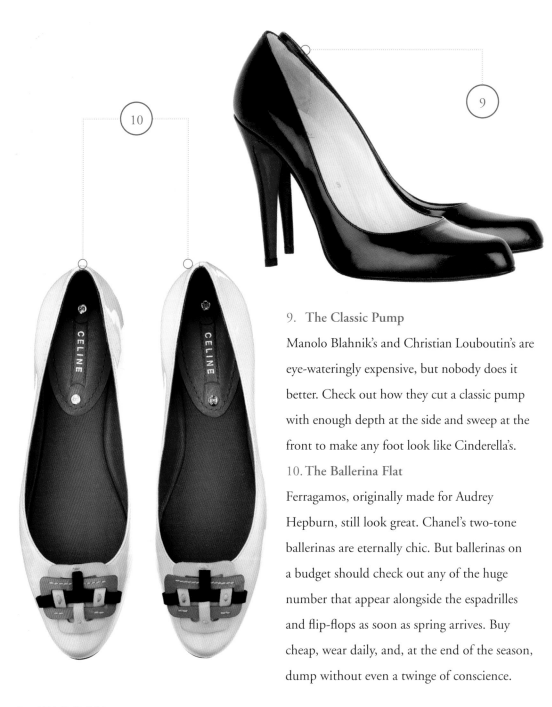

9. **The Classic Pump**

Manolo Blahnik's and Christian Louboutin's are eye-wateringly expensive, but nobody does it better. Check out how they cut a classic pump with enough depth at the side and sweep at the front to make any foot look like Cinderella's.

10. **The Ballerina Flat**

Ferragamos, originally made for Audrey Hepburn, still look great. Chanel's two-tone ballerinas are eternally chic. But ballerinas on a budget should check out any of the huge number that appear alongside the espadrilles and flip-flops as soon as spring arrives. Buy cheap, wear daily, and, at the end of the season, dump without even a twinge of conscience.

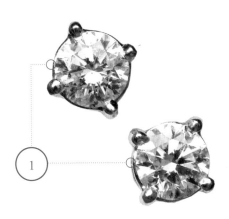

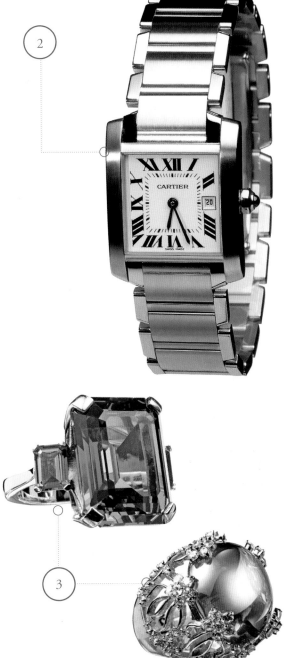

## JEWELRY

### 1. Diamond or Pearl Studs

In the event of a milestone birthday, a landmark anniversary, a promotion, a bonus, or the unexpected arrival of some "mad money," it pays to have a spending plan. In a perfect world, every girl would be born with these in her jewel box. They don't have to be real, and a convincing fake is way better than a teeny specimen that glints only when you squint.

### 2. Cartier Tank Française Watch

The man's version on a woman's wrist is drop-dead sexy.

### 3. The Cocktail Ring

No better way to liven up your little black dress than with a large cocktail ring. Big, semiprecious stones or good look-alikes make a major impact.

## A QUICK COLOR FIX

One great way to bring some old favorites right up to date without busting the budget is to inject some color. If your wardrobe majors in dark-colored classics or trusty neutrals that are still looking too good for a time-out, see how a simple pop of color could help. Experiment with inexpensive additions such as scarves, T-shirts, and belts before you graduate to major color purchases.

- Brown is beautiful with pink and rich with royal blue. Khaki looks softly luxurious with a tawny brown.

- Navy and brown look great together.

- Don't worry if your look doesn't match exactly. Mismatching looks modern. Odd color combinations are cool.

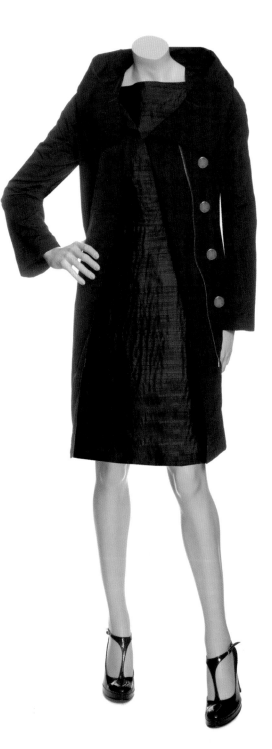

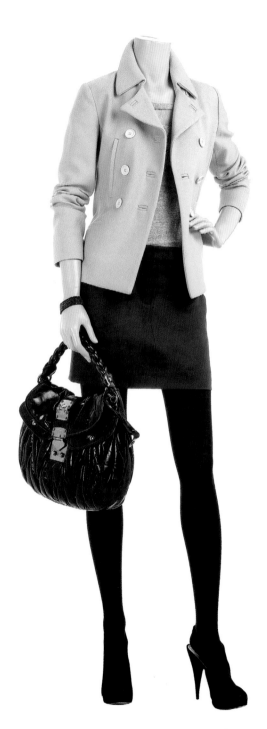

- Make dark classics modern with some offbeat color styling. Check out what a chartreuse tank, a fuchsia scarf, or an orange belt could do for your navy, black, or gray suit.

- Try accenting white or black looks with clear, eye-popping colors: aqua blue or cherry red. Winter white is a real winner. A slightly off-white winter coat is a great investment as the nights draw in.

- When making color statements, know when to stop. Wear a red dress and matching lipstick, but ditch the red shoes. One hot statement is enough.

- New to brights? Choose a matte fabric until you're ready to shine. (Only when you are sure they work for you should you try them in sparkly, shiny, or glossy versions.)

- Your business bag doesn't have to be black or brown. Consider going for a color that makes more of a statement. Lime green, scarlet, or orange, anyone?

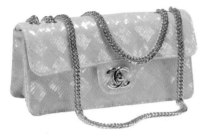

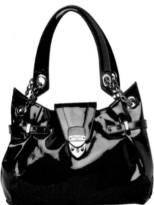

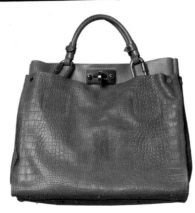

BLACK

There's a reason fashion folk wear black—it's so easy. But be careful about resorting to an all-black wardrobe just because you think it's the key to carefree chic. It will look dreary and bland, not sharp and chic, if you don't loosen things up with texture.

- A black shift and opaque black tights could look great with a charcoal gray or claret cardigan, or a white trench coat.

- A black pencil skirt and black shirt or lightweight sweater will benefit from the briefest glimpse of a white shirt or jewelry at the neck and fine mesh tights instead of thick black ones.

- Black frames and slims, but is also hard on pale complexions, dull in bright sunlight, and visually heavy. If you want to appear slimmer, try using black in the trouble zones (hips, legs, torso, arms, or bust) and freshen up the rest with color.

- If your complexion really can't take black, go for a tone under black: charcoal gray, chocolate brown, navy blue.

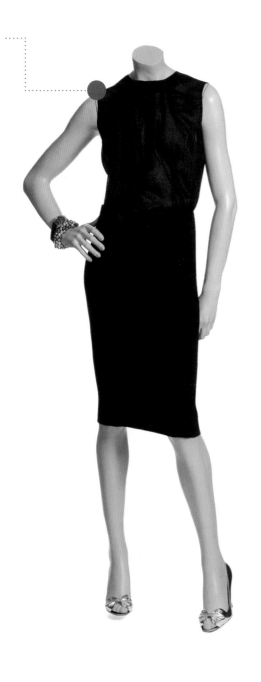

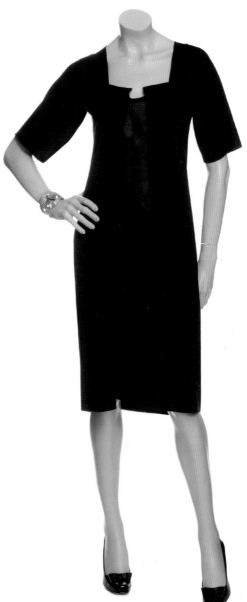

• Black doesn't have to go with black or navy with navy. Mixing the two often looks much more sophisticated.

## NEUTRALS

You know your neutrals work for you but
suspect you need to break out of the beige,
black, and navy blue rut. You and your
neutrals probably have a very good thing
going. Don't be hasty. It might simply be
time to reassess.

- A camel cardigan in a classic style will
  lighten up a whole wardrobe of black
  basics. Camel and beige work on black or
  honey-colored girls but make pale
  redheads and brunettes look ill. If you're
  too pale to wear them, try them from the
  waist down and with black next to your
  face. Nothing beats a slim camel skirt
  and black polo neck.

- Camel and gray are always a chic
  color combination.

- A beige reptile-skin shoe is neutral but
  not boring and will liven up anything
  from jeans to a cocktail dress.

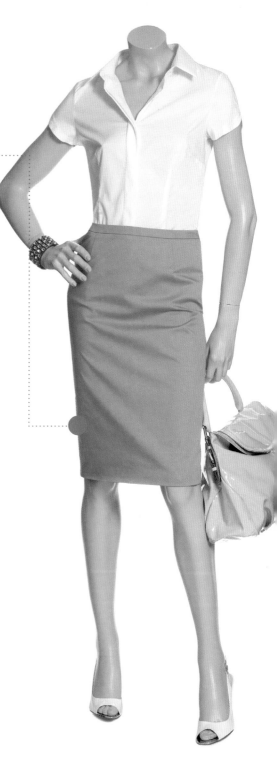

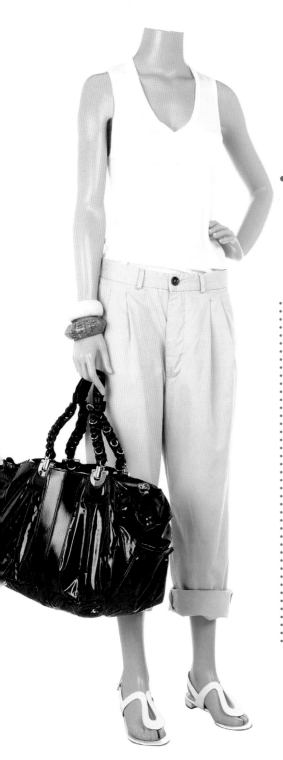

- Hip-slung khakis and a figure-skimming T-shirt, shell, or singlet are modern, casual sexy classics for any age.

# 4

FIGURE

## F L A T T E R Y

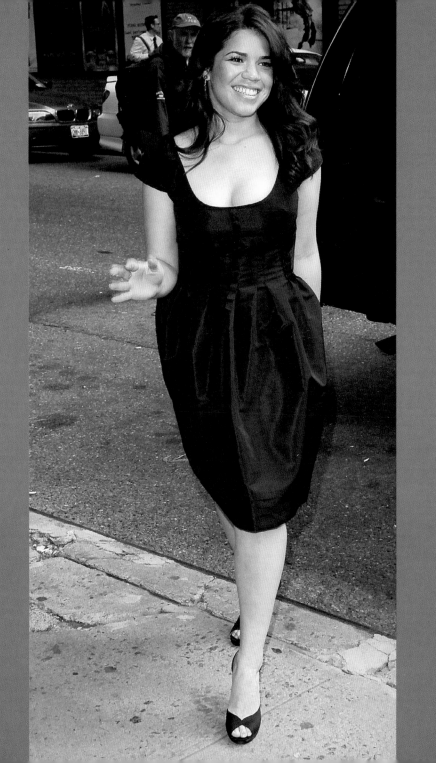

CRUCIAL TO JACKIE KENNEDY'S STYLE LEGACY
WAS HER ABILITY TO EDIT AND CULTIVATE
HER STYLE **ATTRIBUTES—**ASSETS AND FLAWS ALIKE.
**SHE HID HER IMPERFECT TEETH**
WITH A DEMURE SMILE **AND CHOSE HER CLOTHING**
**TO MAXIMIZE** WHAT SHE THOUGHT
**WAS A LESS** THAN IDEAL BODY.

Annette Tapert

DO YOU LOVE YOUR BODY? This question usually prompts a tirade about what is less than perfect. Some "flaws" can be changed; between self-discipline and surgery there are many options. Others cannot. Happily, many of the world's most memorable women have turned their "flaws" into their trademarks. Would Cindy Crawford have been quite so fabulous without her mole? Would Lauren Hutton be so gorgeous with perfectly fixed teeth? Can you imagine Jennifer Lopez without that butt, Kate Moss without her elfin frame, a size-zero Oprah? Enough said!

Make a promise to yourself, today. Accept the things you can't change, no matter how many inches, bulges, or unwanted curves you imagine come between you and perfection. Confidence and knowing what suits you are what matters when it comes to style.

THERE'S NO SUCH THING **AS A PLAIN WOMAN.**
**EVERYONE HAS ATTRACTIVE POINTS,** SO MY ADVICE IS
TO ACCENTUATE **YOUR BEST ASSETS.**

Dita Von Teese

## FIRST THINGS FIRST: KNOW WHAT IS FABULOUS FOR YOU

Try on the clothes that make you feel really good. How does your body look inside them? Work out what it is about your body that makes those clothes look so good.

- What are you always complimented on? (Beautiful neck and shoulders, great cleavage, good legs, graceful arms, great butt?) This is what you should accentuate. Never hide these attributes unless the weather turns nasty.
- Play to your strengths:
  - You have good legs: wear skirts.
  - You have a small waist: wear belts.
  - You have a great bust: ditch the billowing shirts.
  - Great face, bad figure: use accessories that draw attention to your face.
- Find out what colors light up your face, bring out the color of your eyes, and flatter your hair and wear them—all the time.

- Know your list of colors, fabrics, shapes, and lengths to look out for. If you're easily distracted, write everything down and keep it on hand when you're out shopping.

## HOW TO FIND THE BEST FIT

In the changing room, make sure shirts and jackets don't pinch across the back of your arms and shoulders. But don't overdo it—tailored clothes that are too loose are as powerful a figure killer as those that pinch. If you're small, you look overwhelmed. If you're not small, you look bigger than you are. A garment is tailored to perfection for you if it skims, never squeezes, the body. The right size will minimize, but even a gentle squeeze will make you look bigger than you are.

Never forget: Body shapers do a good job of lifting and smoothing. Don't be afraid to use them to achieve that perfect fit. But always work within the limits of the Lycra. If you ask too much of your control panties, you'll have bulges where nature never intended them to be.

## SOME POINTERS
## FOR THE FULL-FIGURED

- If you have a curvy figure, avoid fussy details at the neck, including scarves, big bows, and frilly collars.

- Heavy arms need long sleeves that preferably skim, never grip the flesh. Cap sleeves accentuate flabby upper arms.

- You can wear short sleeves even if your arms are less than perfectly toned; just make sure the sleeves aren't tight.

- A narrow tunic-style top worn over slim pants will create an illusion of overall slimness and draw the eye away from your tummy. (No smocks, please!)

- Flat-front trousers smooth and reduce while pleat-fronted trousers billow and add inches.

- If you want to camouflage your tummy, go for blouson-shape tops that settle low on your hip bones, but stick to drapey fabrics that move, such as jersey or crepe. The same shape in a bulky fabric, such as wool or velour, will look lumpy. Keep the bottom half slim to balance everything out.

- Wide, straight-legged trousers will camouflage heavy legs. Make sure the hem breaks on the top of your shoes. A hem that hovers above your shoes will add width.

- Never *ever* choose pants with an elasticized waist over a tailored pair. Tailored pants will slim and control your shape. Elasticized pants will let it all hang out.

- Asymmetry, particularly draping, is a great way to smooth out unwanted curves. A bias-cut dress in a substantial fabric, such as a good jersey, is a good tummy tamer. All soft A-lines are good tummy flatterers.

- Go for a sharp shoulder and a curve at the waist. Dressing from head to toe in big, baggy clothes looks awful.

- Full-figured women look best in long drop earrings. Button clips and big, spherical studs are like punctuation marks that accentuate roundness.

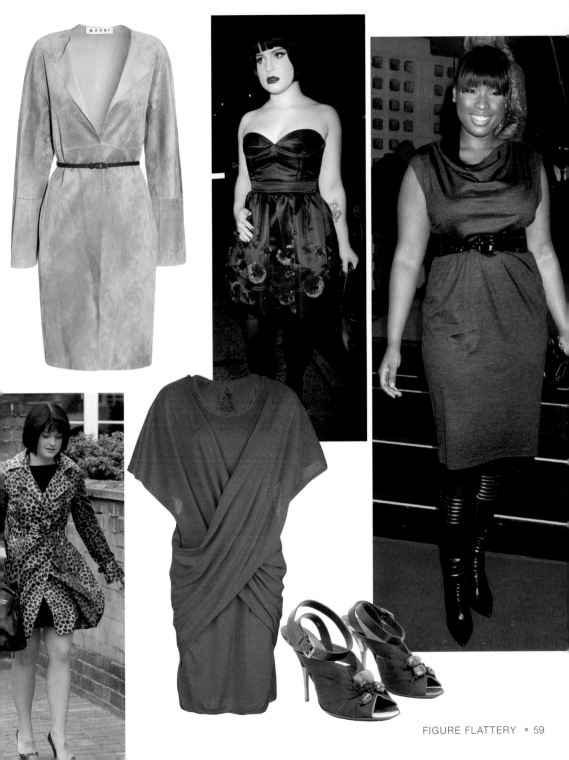

## SOME POINTERS FOR PETITES

- Petites wearing horizontal lines are shortened even further. It cuts them in half. Treat bright belts with the same caution.

- Petite women should avoid wearing clothes at their natural waistline. Drop-waist trousers, skirts, and dresses look sharper. If you lower the waistline even by an inch, the torso will look longer and narrower.

- Skinny sleeves set in a high armhole are the most flattering.

- Slim pants cropped at the ankle will add valuable inches to your leg with either flat or high-heeled shoes.

- A neatly tailored shift or bias-cut dress and mid-heeled pumps are your default position for fail-safe figure flattery.

- Dresses, rather than separates, will lengthen petites.

- Empire waistlines (ones that fit under the bust) are also great lengtheners.

- Petites, particularly curvy ones, look better in skirts rather than trousers.

- Petites can wear longer skirts, but make sure the proportion is spot-on. Heels are mandatory, and a simple, slim top will add height. Avoid very full skirts that hit anywhere below the knee.

- Knee-length coats are dramatic and slimming for everyone, but you'll look even better if you go slightly shorter.

- Big shoulder pads and stiffly tailored clothes are death to a petite woman, particularly if she is also fuller-figured. Soft lines and fluid fabrics are much more flattering.

- Petites with boyish figures should avoid knee-high boots. Mid-calf is better.

- A very short woman in very high heels looks ridiculous. A medium-height heel is best.

- Petite women who have the arms of jackets shortened to fit should also check if the width also needs attention to keep the proportion right. The same goes for trouser legs. Short and wide is not a good look for anyone trying to add height.

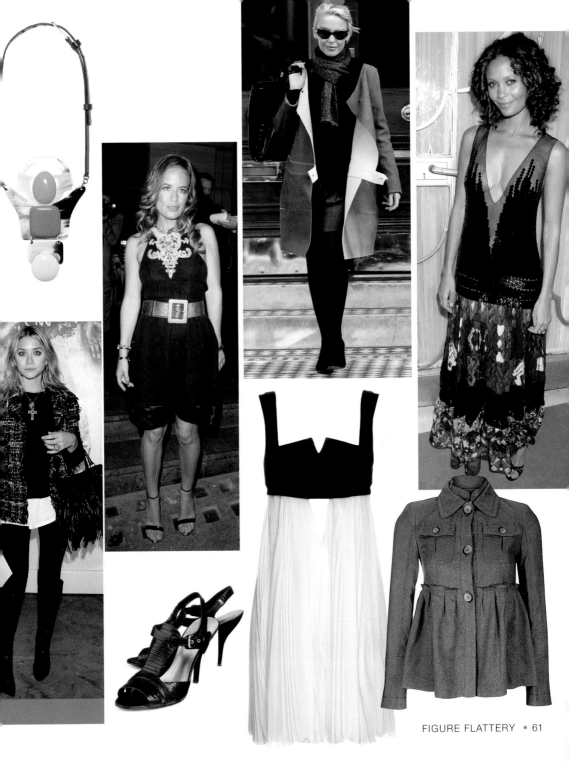

## SOME POINTERS
## FOR BOYISH FIGURES

- If you have a very boyish figure and no waist, a big belt slung low on the hips will often create a more convincing illusion of curves than a belt cinched tightly right on the waist. And a shirt knotted on the waist will give as much definition as a belt.

- Stick with dark belts. A colorful belt makes all waists look wider.

- For women with no curves who want some *va va voom*, the waist is a pivotal point. A top with volume tucked into a figure-skimming skirt will create sexy curves where none exist. What you lose in height with volume can be countered with a wide belt on the waist.

- If you have no bottom, avoid tight, straight skirts. Go for an A-line instead.

- A full skirt will work wonders. The volume of fabric swishing around makes you walk and hold yourself differently. Shoes with a heel, even a low kitten heel, will do the same. It's not what you haven't got, it's how you carry it that matters. (What you lose in height with a full skirt can be countered with a wide belt on the waist.)

- Women with boyish figures can really carry off clothes cut in heavier fabrics and ought to experiment with tweeds, corduroys, and heavy twills.

- Pleated trousers will give you curves if you have no hips, but to be able to carry them off you must be tall (at least 5'7") and have a flat tummy. If you don't, flat-front trousers are best, every time.

- Extreme skirts: Ballerina skirts, ball skirts, gypsy skirts, and long A-line skirts are chic on you. Just wear them as simply as possible. Try them with a boat-necked leotard that shows off your collarbone, or a white singlet top. And go for the cinch with a great belt to define your waist. A cardigan with a billowing skirt is chic if you're tall, but make sure the sleeves stop just below the elbow (push them up if necessary) to avoid a droopy look.

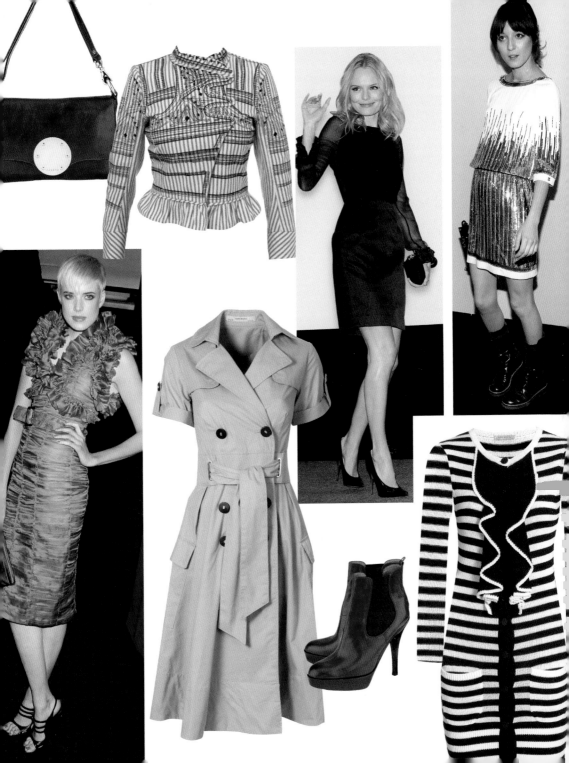

## SOME POINTERS FOR PEAR SHAPES

- Never try to make a straight line out of ample curves. Voluminous clothes that drop from the shoulder will not camouflage extra pounds; they'll make you look shapeless and bigger than you are. Try to go in and out a bit: thinner at the waist and narrower at the knee.

- The alternative is a neutral-colored and figure-skimming silhouette (such as a tailored dress or tailored shell and pants) topped with a loose-cut knee-length coat left open. Don't be afraid to make statements with a coat that has strong color or rich texture.

- Pear-shaped women should never cinch their waists. Instead, try raising your waistline (it'll make your legs look longer and smooth out the silhouette) or lowering it. Cardigans that fit loosely buttoned to just above your waist and with the top buttons left undone raise waistlines. A softly tailored shirt worn unbuttoned over a T-shirt the same way

will also do this. A belt anchoring a hip-length top with easy volume (never tight) will lower your waist, and the gentle volume will rebalance your proportions.

- You can use hipster belts on wide hips to create interest under a jacket. If your belt buckle attracts attention, make sure your stomach and bosom don't.

- An off-shoulder neckline, or seaming across the upper back of a dress or shirt that reaches from shoulder to shoulder, will minimize the waist by widening the shoulders.

- A great hip-minimizing outfit is a fingertip-length jacket, nipped in slightly at the waist (so it's not too boxy), worn over straight-legged trousers or a skirt in a fluid fabric, with high heels. The slight flare of boot-leg trousers or a soft A-line skirt balances full hips. A figure-skimming rather than figure-hugging cut is more flattering. Wearing heels under your trousers will further boost the slimming effect.

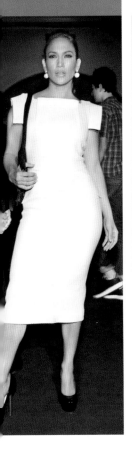

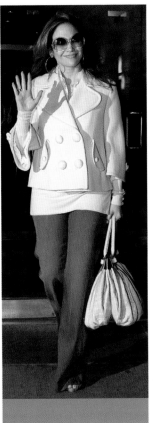

I'VE GOT A STOMACH
**AS WELL AS A BEHIND.**
**AND I MEAN—WELL,** YOU CAN'T
PULL IT IN BOTH WAYS, **CAN YOU? . . .**
**I'VE MADE IT A RULE**
TO PULL IN MY STOMACH
**AND LET MY BEHIND**
LOOK AFTER ITSELF.

Agatha Christie, *The Dressmaker's Doll*

- The classic alternative, the three-quarter length jacket that hits just above the knee, has honestly had its day. It has become such a style cliché among pear-shaped women that it advertises wide hips almost as much as a short jacket would. A good alternative is a wrap jacket (as long as it doesn't cinch too tightly at the waist) that hits at thigh length. Softer cardigan styles or shirt jackets are great options for casual situations. Very structured jackets can work, but often look best left open over wide hips.

- Another great look is the slim-fitting (tunic-style) top over straight-cut trousers that skim the body. This line creates an illusion of overall slimness and draws the eye away from your tummy. Make sure the trousers are flat-front, and avoid cuffs.

- Pockets with flaps and trousers with pleats make very few women look good. Flapless pockets and flat-front trousers look better on anyone. But be careful: big patch pockets also add width. The only place they really look good is on the back of your jeans.

- The way suede skirts and pants can firm a flabby hip is one of the style wonders of the world.

- If you have ample hips, avoid miniskirts at all costs. They focus attention right where you don't want it.

- Dressing in one fabric from head to toe does nothing for a curvy body. Opt for separates and experiment with textures rather than colors to create interest. (Remember: shiny textures expand, matte minimizes.)

- Pear-shaped women can look fantastic in jeans. Go for stretch and a figure-skimming fit rather than loose cut.

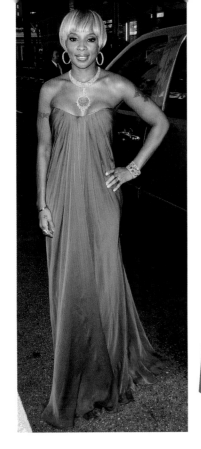

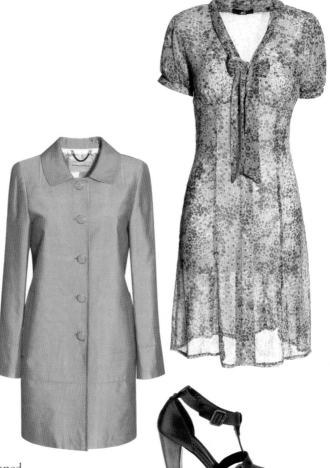

- A common mistake among pear-shaped women looking to make fashion impact is to go for the big-shouldered look. Don't! Big shoulders are really not the best counterbalance in this case. Shoulder pads that veer inches away from your actual shoulder line just look sloppy. Your natural shoulder line, sharply defined, looks better.

- Try using bare flesh to divert attention. Shoulders are one of the most effective decoys of all. A bare back will also minimize wide hips. But be careful. Big-bosomed women should never go backless without adequate support.

## HOW TO DRESS A BIG BUST (AND MAKE THE MOST OF NO BUST AT ALL): DIVERSION TACTICS FOR HANDLING THE MOST DANGEROUS CURVES

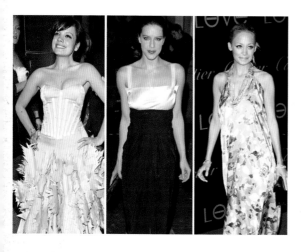

### Diversion #1: Shoulders

When making the most of a glorious bust—or even a nonexistent one—remember that your shoulders are key. Keep shoulder pads sharply defined, and never veer off your natural shoulder line. Naked shoulders will divert attention from a large bust, but never go strapless without adequate support. You'll just look shapeless.

### Diversion #2: Neckline

Your neckline is a powerful proportion adjuster. Next time you reach for a cover-up, remember that V-necks and open collars slim and lengthen the torso, so open up a little. A collar is one of the most versatile style weapons. It can lighten and pull your entire look together and frame your face like a great hat (but without the fuss). For example, a crisp white collar, worn with a black or gray V-neck or round-neck cardigan, makes this most comfortable of all knitwear look sharp, not sloppy. Try a square neckline for a change. If it fits properly, this shape looks great on an ample bust.

Halter necks were made for flat-chested women. A halter in a slightly drapey fabric will work untold wonders. They rarely work for big-bosomed women because it's so hard to get adequate support.

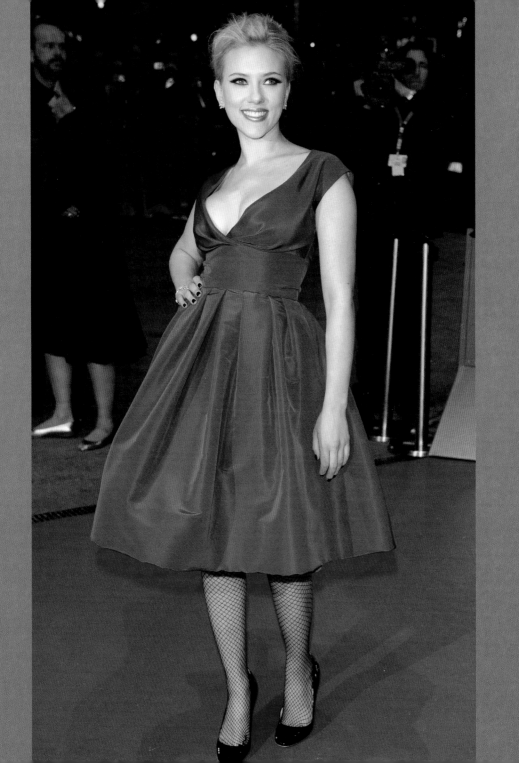

## If Your Bust Is Large

For starters: Never hide a great bust in big shirts. If your bust is bigger than you'd like it to be, draping it in voluminous layers is not going to make it any smaller. In fact, with all that fabric flapping about, you're in treacherous fashion territory. What you think is a clever disguise is drawing attention right where you don't want it. You should be aiming for "trim silhouette," not "galleon in full sail." There are three cardinal rules:

### Rule 1

A well-made, properly fitted bra is never an extravagance, no matter how much it costs. Underwear that gives you the support you need will minimize and shape the way nothing else can, short of surgery. A bra that minimizes by squashing you can create a quadraboob that's visible even through tailored clothes.

### Rule 2

A body-skimming silhouette is kinder than a baggy one. If that leaves you feeling too exposed, top it with a looser layer, but leave the slim layer underneath visible. Try a fine-knit sweater under a shirt jacket or a fine-knit cardigan over a tailored dress.

### Rule 3

Avoid high-necked sweaters. Unless you have enough chutzpah to carry off the curvaceous cling à la Anita Ekberg, you're in danger of ending up with the matron's monoboob.

## TRY THIS FOR DOWNSIZING

- A dark top (solid colors, not prints) worn with a lighter-colored bottom half will minimize a large bust.

- If you have a bust larger than a B cup, skinny tops with breast pockets (especially with flaps) are a big no-no.

- Avoid dressing an ample bust in tunic tops: they will drop straight down from a full bust and make you look pregnant.

- Don't always try to hide or minimize a large bust. Show it off once in a while, but with proper support. A corset top or dress with built-in bustier will look great.

- The best sweaters are V-necks that aren't cut too low, sleeveless tanks, and fitted, long-sleeved polo necks. Crew necks and

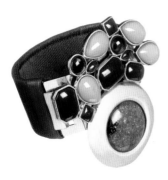

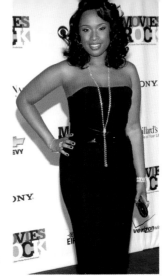

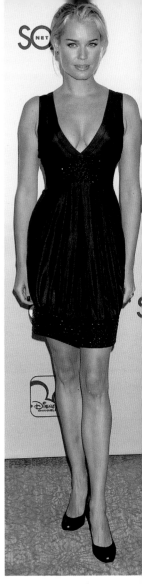

buttoned-up cardigans are the least flattering shapes.

- Slim your torso by experimenting with a tailored top and full trousers.
- If you are slim below the waist, experiment with trousers or skirts in colors that are lighter or brighter than your top. A solid dark-colored top worn with a lighter bottom half is a great minimizing trick.
- Dresses with empire waistlines are out, but a tailored shift with a square neckline will look amazing.
- Don't wear wide belts or waistbands that shorten the upper body. They are sure to draw attention to a large bust.
- Go for bracelets and earrings: any piece that draws attention away from your bust.
- Avoid dangling pendants and long ropes of beads.

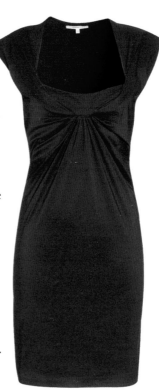

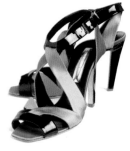

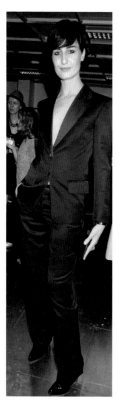

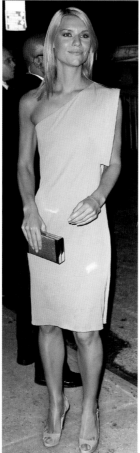

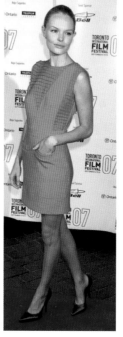

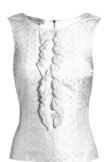

### If Your Bust Is Small

- Pleats, ruffles, and gathering add volume to a small bust in a chic way. Try a softly pleated halter top or blouse. If you have a boyish figure the volume on top can also create the illusion of a waist.

- Bustiers create curves for women without them.

- Padded push-up bras that squeeze you together are not the best way to boost a small bust. Try a balconette bra instead, with padding, if necessary. The wide-set straps give shape uplift as well as a broader line across the shoulders. It's a much prettier effect.

## SHOULDERS: EVERY WOMAN'S SECRET STYLE WEAPON

### Dressed

Make sure shoulders fit properly. They should define your shape or, at most, sharpen it. Shoulder pads that veer inches away from your actual shoulder line look sloppy.

### Undressed

Bare shoulders are one of fashion's most effective decoys. They will counter a straight waist and minimize wide hips in an instant. And they are one of the last parts of a woman's anatomy to show her age.

### Narrow or Sloping Shoulders

- If you have sloping or narrow shoulders, a boatneck will better boost your shoulder line than big shoulder pads.
- Coats with defined shoulders will look best. The trench is made for you, but make sure the shoulders sit neatly.
- Avoid drawing attention to the center line of the body with neckties, long scarves, long necklaces, or tight tops: These all emphasize the fact that your hips are wider than your shoulders.

### Wide Shoulders

A definite fashion asset. If they make you feel self-conscious, avoid cutaway armholes and stretchy tube tops.

## NECKLINE

Your neckline is your upper torso's framing device. Here are six neckline secrets that won't let you down:

1. Square necklines really set off small faces.
2. Polo necks emphasize a striking chin and jaw.
3. Boat and slash-necks are a gift for any woman trying to minimize from the waist down and maximize her shoulders.
4. Halters are great for showing off gorgeous shoulders and distracting the eye from the hips.
5. V-necks and open collars slim and lengthen the torso.
6. If you have a very skinny neck, avoid very delicate necklaces. Go instead for a chunky choker or a high collar that accentuates your neck's length.

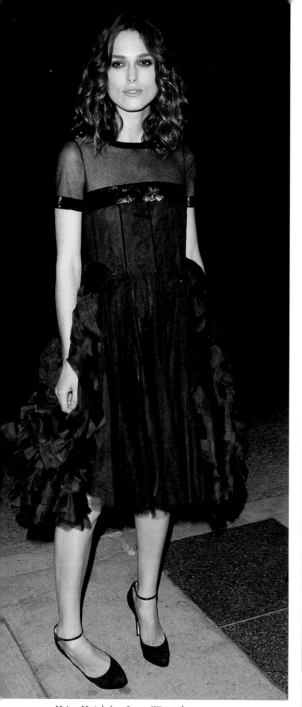

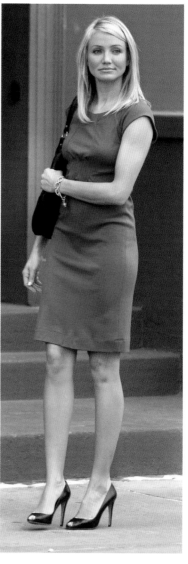

## UNIVERSAL STYLE TRUTH

Straighten up! Nothing is more eye-catching than a woman who walks tall.

*Cameron Diaz: Short-Waisted*

*Keira Knightley: Long-Waisted*

## THE WAIST

*First—Are You Short- or Long-Waisted?*

- Short waist = torso is short in relation to your legs.
- Long waist = torso is long in relation to your legs.
  - If you have a short waist, avoid cropped jackets, high-waisted skirts, or empire lines. Instead, try a long top with a short skirt. A slim sweater worn untucked over a skirt will lengthen your body.
  - Short-waisted women should steer clear of flamboyant buckles or wide, brightly colored belts. If your hips are narrow, a low-slung belt will lengthen your waist.
  - Long-waisted women should aim for shorter tops with a long line bottom half. A shirt, knotted just above your waist, will do the same trick.
  - Use a belt to move your waist. Short-waisted women should try matching their belt with the color of their top. Long-waisted women should go for a belt the color of their skirt or trousers.

## A WORD ON HEMLINES

Hem lengths are no longer dictated by fashion. You can wear what suits you and look great no matter what look is "hot."

- The most flattering hemline is right at the knee. It hovers between the obvious and the frumpy. For most people, the right length is just below the crinkly bit of the knee. However, if your knees are great, you get to break the rule and bare them. Just be honest with yourself. Good knees are an endangered species.
- Great knees or no, don't commit what, in Paris, is considered to be the cardinal fashion sin and wear miniskirts just because you have great legs. (Coco Chanel called the miniskirted over-thirties "old little girls.") It's rare that a mature face fits this girly hem length's mood.
- If you've found the length that works best for you, stick to it. As long as you're completely honest with yourself, then no matter what a fashion expert may tell you, the choice between a knee-length

skirt that you know suits you and a miniskirt that is simply fashionable is obvious. Same goes for trousers. If cropped trousers shorten your leg, don't wear them just because everyone else is. In any case, each length requires a different shoe and jacket. Who has the time?

## LEGS

- Pale-colored hose will thicken any leg. Dark colors will slim and lengthen.

- Heavily patterned or textured tights also add bulk. Wear them only if you want the extra width. Even hose with a linear pattern will add weight, because the straight lines wobble over bulges.

- If you must do texture, make it a fine fishnet. If you must do color, make them berry tones, burgundy, mossy greens, or charcoals instead of orange, scarlet, yellow, or royal blue. White tights and bright primary or acid colors look good only on mannequins. High heels instantly make all legs look slimmer.

- Wide or cropped trousers and cuffs shorten all legs. Don't wear them unless you can afford to lose a few inches. If you aren't sure, try wide trousers over high heels.

- Wear stockings that match your shoes, not your skirt. In most cases it looks better and in all cases it lengthens the leg.

- Legs will look longer in sheer, flesh-colored hose and a nude-colored high heel.

- *Never* let footless tights cut you off at the calf. They need to reach at least to where your lower leg gets slimmer.

- Ankle-strap shoes make most ankles look chunky and shorten legs.

- The more open the top of the shoe, the longer the leg line. Ditto when it comes to the back of the shoe. This is why mules look great on just about everyone.

## FIVE WAYS FOR ANYBODY TO ADD HEIGHT

1. A V-neck will always give a torso a few inches and make your neck appear longer. A shirt or single-breasted jacket with narrow lapels is also in this category.

2. Vertical stripes or pinstripes (not too loud or you'll look like Krusty the Clown) slim and lengthen.

3. Try wearing a jacket in a bright or light color over dark navy, black, or brown separates, such as trousers, skirts, even a dark T-shirt.

4. Avoid lots of flounces and frills. Simple, narrow single-breasted suit jackets, three-quarter-length belted coats, long narrow trousers with hems that almost skim the floor worn over high heels, and straight or A-line skirts that hit just below or on the knee are all good. Choose a slim column gown over flamenco ruffles.

5. The easiest way to lengthen your leg is to wear delicate heels, cut low at the side of your foot with a slightly pointed toe. Avoid anything that cuts across your leg at any level, such as calf-high or ankle boots or T-strap shoes. Knee-high boots will lengthen your leg more effectively if they hit the place where your leg goes in under the knee. If you are wearing boots with a skirt, choose hose that match the color of your boots.

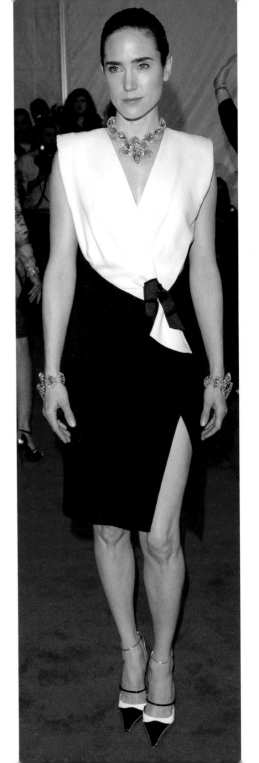

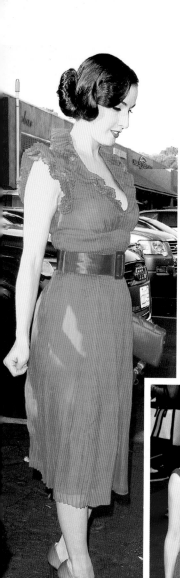

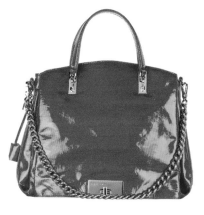

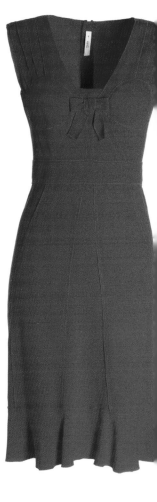

# WHEN IN DOUBT,
## WEAR RED.

Bill Blass

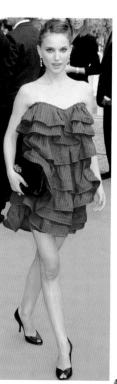

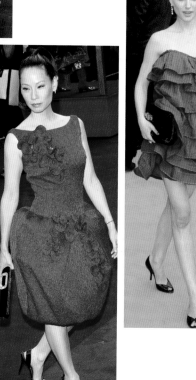

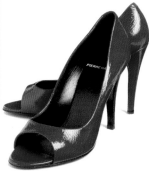

## A WORD ABOUT COLOR

- White adds weight, black reduces.
- Colors that expand your figure instantly are white, yellow, orange, lime green, and almost all shades of pink.
- Colors that camouflage are neutrals and almost all pastels—everything from caramel to ice blue. (For pastel pink, see above.)
- Colors that contain your figure are black, navy, charcoal, dark brown, and gray.
- Any dark color worn head to toe in a clean line will have a dramatically slimming and lengthening effect. Alleviate the dullness by working with textures: matte with shine or knit with woven, for example. Be careful—texture and shine can add weight.
- Consider shiny textures in the same category as light colors and matte the same as dark and use them to highlight or camouflage appropriately. For example, if you want to camouflage a large bust, a (light-colored) skirt with shine and (dark-colored) matte top is for you.
- A solid-colored dress in a fluid fabric that grazes the body is likely to become a favorite.

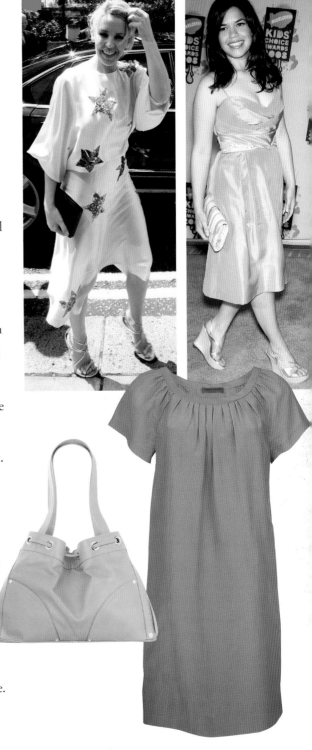

## PRINTS

- Big prints, large polka dots, horizontal stripes (even as texture in knits), and patterned leggings are all fattening.

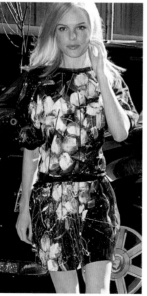

- A small, uniform allover design keeps the eye moving and therefore camouflages lumps and bumps.

- Short figures are flattered by prints with low-contrast (shades of one color) prints. Petites need to avoid busy prints (and all other fussy details) like the plague.

- If you are new to wearing prints, go gently. Beginners are best off choosing something with lower contrast. Soft, floral pastels and dark-toned plaids can be worn by almost anyone, if they're confined to one element of clothing worn with a complementary solid element.

- Unless Christian Lacroix himself is dressing you, stick to one printed item per outfit . . . even if it's shoes.

- Taller bodies can take prints with more contrast.

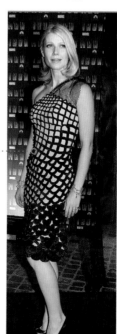

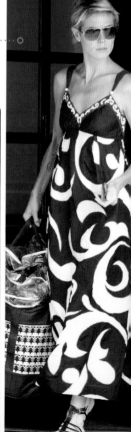

- For most women, prints look better on relaxed styles rather than stretch or sharply tailored styles. Those who are very toned can go for a little stretch or structure, but don't ask a big print to give too much. Those tea roses don't look so good when spread over an ample hip.

- Large florals, bright geometrics, and tropical prints generally look better on the bottom half with an understated and solid color for the top. It's a great look on almost anyone, but it's heaven-sent for those with an ample bust.

- The darker the print's background, the slimmer the look.

- Very boyish figures can handle busy patterns and prints on the top half, as long as they keep the shape simple and balance the effect with a solid-colored bottom half. Pear-shaped women can also go for a print on the top half to draw the eye away from their hips.

- Some ethnic prints are big and great fun. Some look like you bought them at a tourist bazaar. Be wary of the pitfalls and you'll know what's right when you put it on.

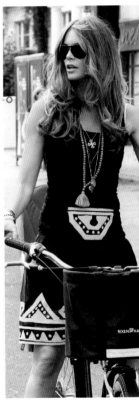

- Full-figured women look best in a print on a fabric that has fluidity. Avoid too much volume, which adds bulk. But as long as it moves, it can look great.

- Animal prints look best if the print looks like the animal it's meant to represent. For example: turquoise and navy are a great color combination. But a turqoise and navy zebra stripe is overwhelming.

# 5

## DRESSING YOUR

A               G               E

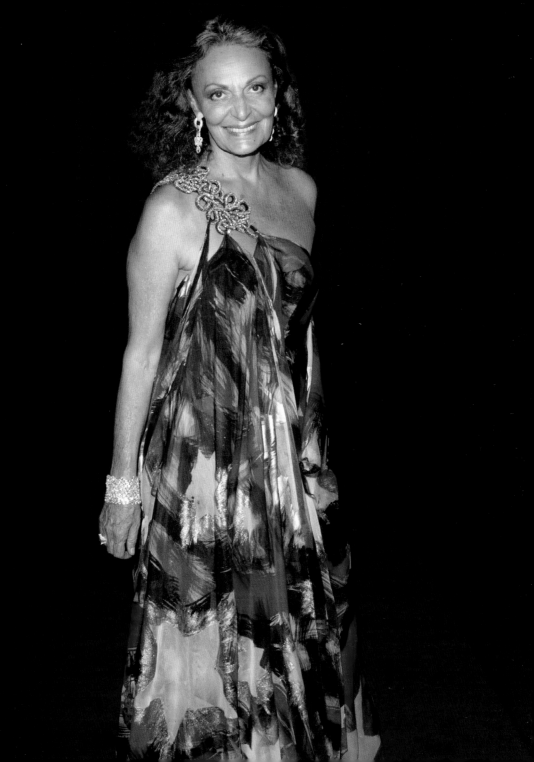

# YOU CAN BE **GORGEOUS AT TWENTY,** CHARMING **AT FORTY, AND IRRESISTIBLE FOR THE REST** OF YOUR LIFE.

Coco Chanel

THERE WAS A TIME not so long ago when a woman over forty could no longer wear trousers, and on anyone over thirty, long hair made you "mutton dressed as lamb." There were rules, and they left you in no doubt about what was right and what was wrong. All questions regarding style had nonnegotiable answers.

At about the same time, if designers decided that miniskirts were in, then miniskirts were what you had to wear. The option, for those with less than lovely legs, was to sit the season out in a kind of style isolation. Past a certain age, you floated off into a fashion wilderness, never again to emerge from a shroud of tweeds and sensible shoes.

Hurrah! Those days are gone. Designers no longer dictate. They propose. The rules are relaxed. We have choices, which should be great but often isn't. No one is going to tell you that a puffball skirt is wrong for you—you're just supposed to know.

Sometimes it's easy. If fashion is all about the miniskirt and you have less than great legs, it's a no-brainer: You go for something else. But if you have great legs that just happen to be circling forty and have looked great in miniskirts at least twice already in the past twenty years, what then? It's a thorny issue, as much about how you feel as how your body looks and whether your face fits.

Appropriateness is not the answer. It can kill a great look faster than a footballer's wife.

It can send a fantastic-looking forty-year-old straight into middle age and make a twenty-year-old going for her first job look like a dull man in drag. It's an outdated concept in a world where women look and feel younger than ever. When you see more and more women in their sixties scoring as highly on fashion's scale of cool as women in their thirties, and not looking at all ridiculous, that's progress, not a reason to go *tut-tut*.

And as more and more women become powerful role models in formal workplaces, it's less necessary for young women to dress in dreary suits to be taken seriously. Whatever your age, you must always buy what makes you look best.

So, are there any new rules that can help us steer a path through what used to be black-and-white and is now just endless shades of gray?

## IF YOU **DON'T BREAK THE RULES,** YOU DON'T HAVE **ANY FUN.**

Anita Pallenberg

### TWENTIES

Clearly, the younger you are, the greater the risks you can take and the more likely you are to pull it all off. Experiment with the hottest trends. The only limits are those set by your figure (a muffin top rules bare midriffs out at any age) and your lifestyle (microminis will undermine your credibility in most offices, but so will those too-dull suits). Apart from that, experiment with everything that appeals to you.

## **VAIN TRIFLES** AS THEY SEEM, **CLOTHES . . . CHANGE OUR VIEW** OF THE WORLD **AND THE WORLD'S** VIEW OF US.

Virginia Woolf

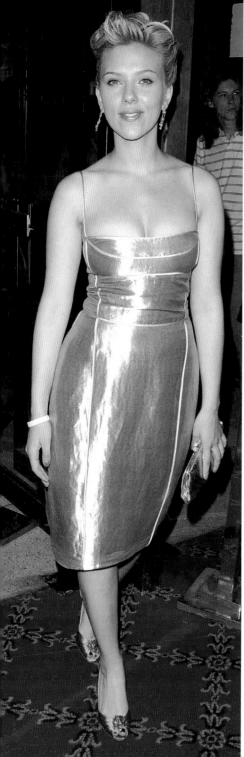

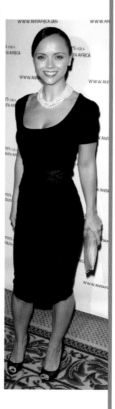

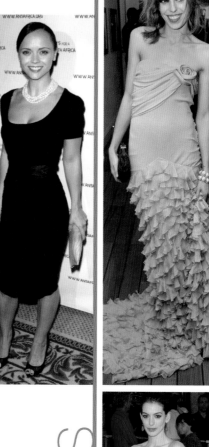

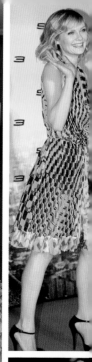

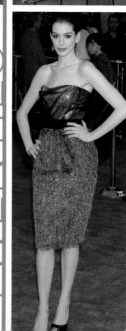

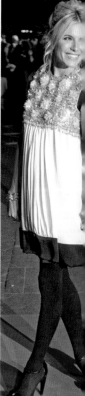

TWENTIES

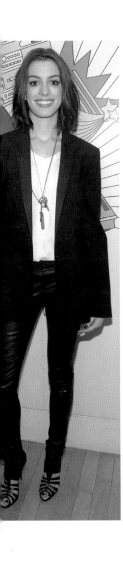

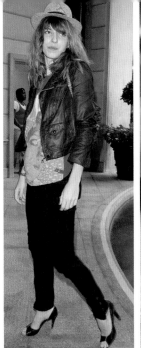

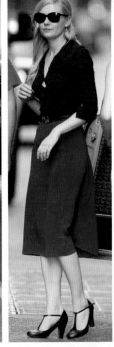

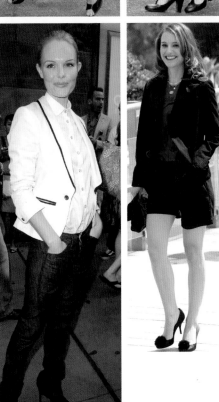

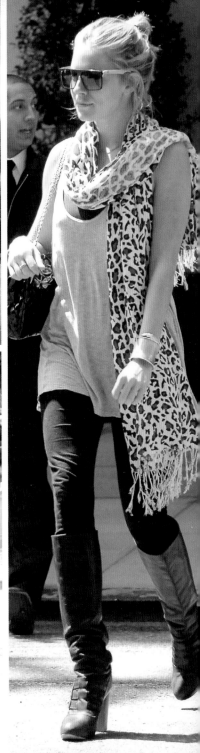

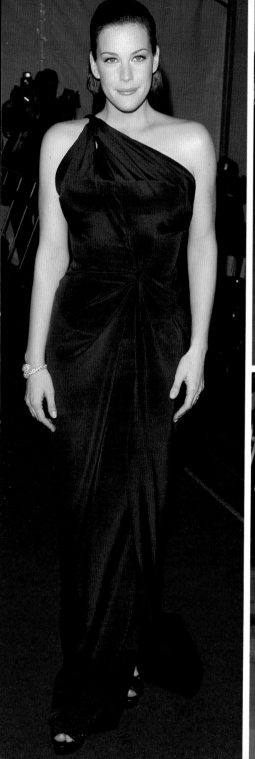

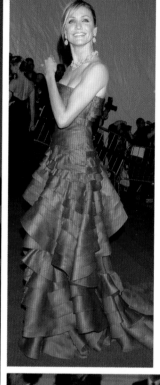

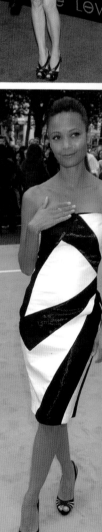

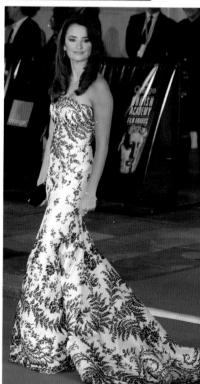

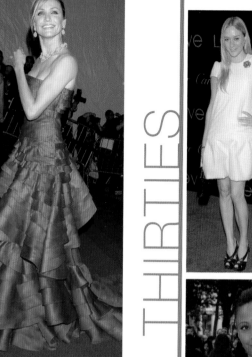

## THIRTIES

Now is when your own style really emerges.
You know your body and should have
an idea of what makes it look good and
what shape does you no favors at all. As
time goes on, you'll face more and more
of these style challenges. Self-knowledge is
a wonderful thing: a secret weapon, more
effective than surgery.

It may be time to reassess some old
favorites: do the low-slung, thong-baring
pants still work for you? Is your clubbing
gear still a useful evening staple, when
perhaps you find you spend more time
socializing in restaurants than nightclubs? It
may also be time to consider stuff you never
thought belonged to your look before: you
may suddenly see sex appeal in tailoring and
feel a yearning that makes a cashmere coat
an absolute essential. You'll undoubtedly
still pick from among the season's trends,
snapping up what makes you look great,
but by now you should know enough about
what's right for you to leave the rest alone.

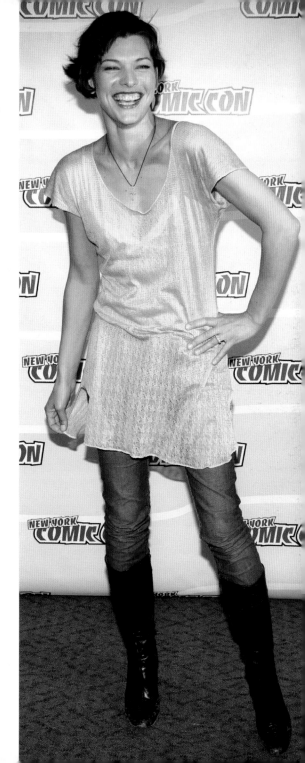

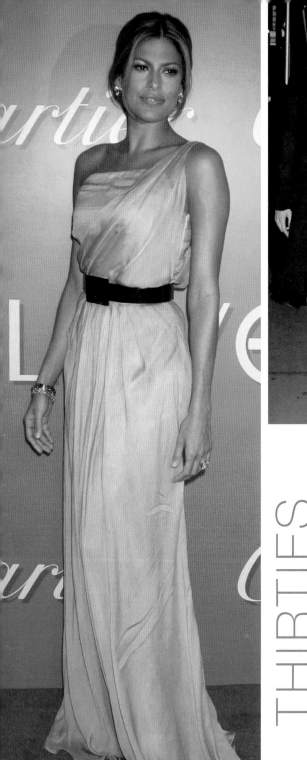
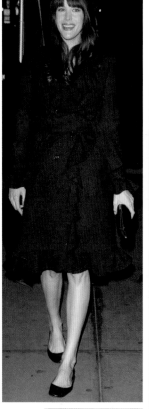
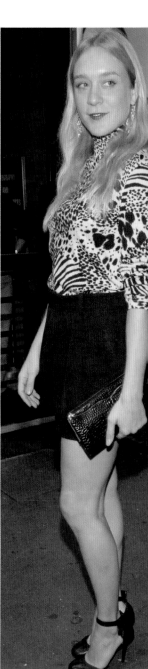
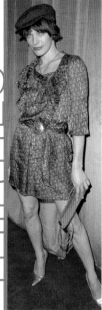

THIRTIES

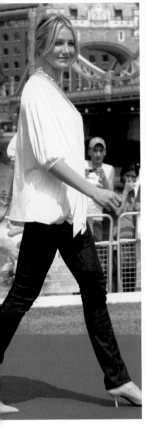

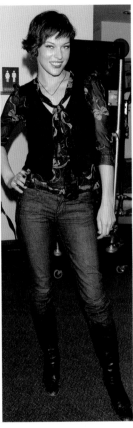

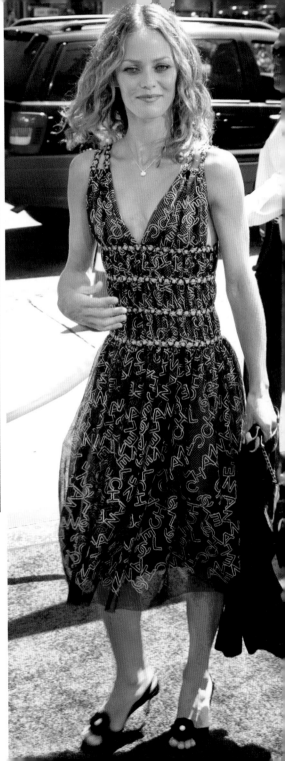

Here is where you stop being a slave to
fashion and start to feel comfortable with
your own style. If you have your body and
your style worked out well enough, you
should begin to find your clothes crossing
several seasons with ease, so aim for
quality that lasts.

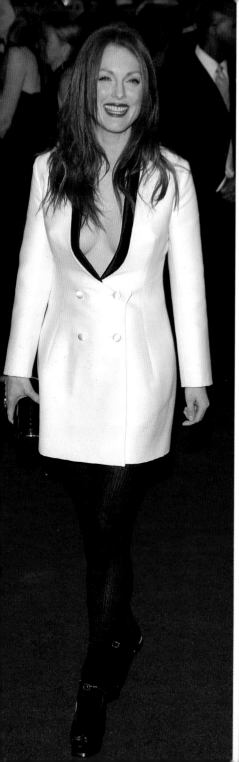

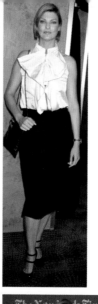

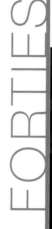

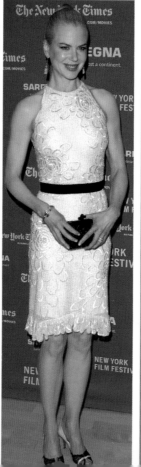

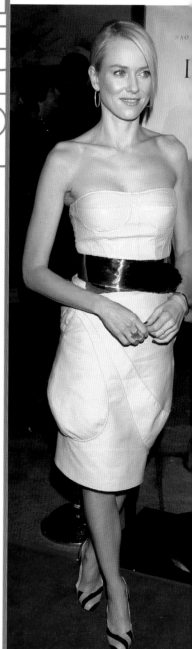

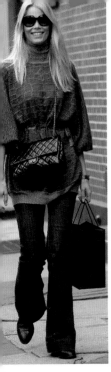
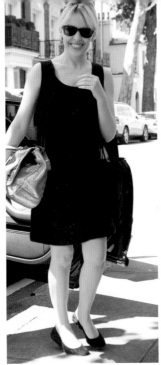
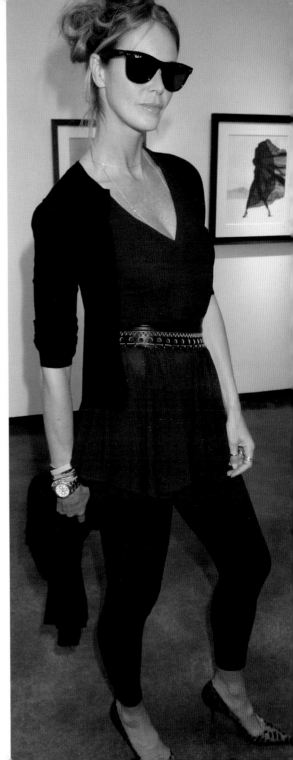

## FORTIES

By now your wardrobe should be 60:40—60 percent investment (which doesn't mean dull, it means well-made pieces that you love and plan to keep for a long time) and 40 percent of the moment. Never rule out new trends if they're really you. But liberal interpretations of the new season's looks and versions once or twice removed from the catwalk originals are likely to be a better bet. Got a great body and ready for fashion's passion for sheer? Try delicate lace or chiffon tops over camouflaging underpinnings and

AT FORTY, WOMEN USED TO EXCHANGE YOUTH
FOR ELEGANCE, POISE, AND MYSTERIOUS ALLURE,
AN EVOLUTION THAT LEFT THEM UNDAMAGED.
NOW THEY MEASURE THEMSELVES AGAINST
THE VERY YOUNG WITH DEFENSES THAT CAN
ONLY BE DESCRIBED AS RIDICULOUS.

Coco Chanel

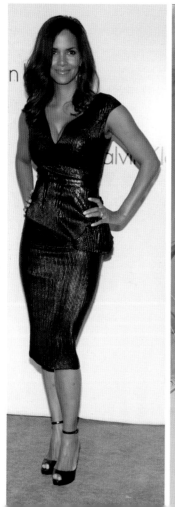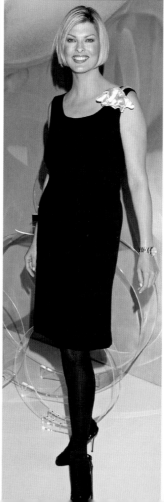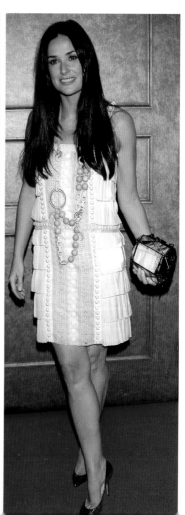

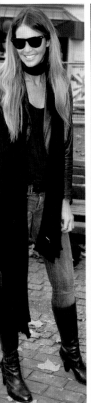

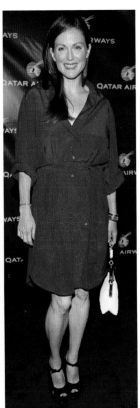

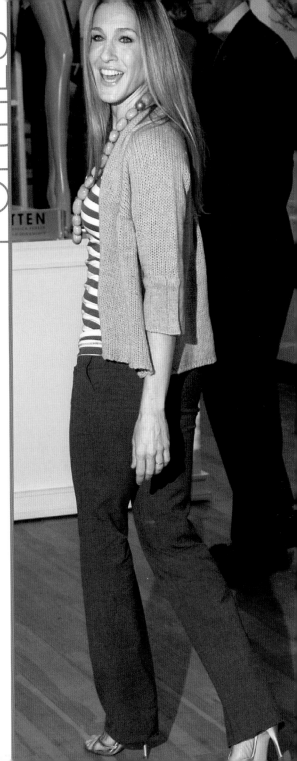

pass on the opportunity to bare all. And be wary of anything too prim. A tweed jacket may look better on a twentysomething (the irony of coltish youth in middle-aged classics is hot) than on a fortysomething (where it can look plain stuffy). Finally, watch your weight. Being underweight can often look worse than a few extra pounds at this age. It may still be entirely possible not to be too rich, but you certainly can be too thin.

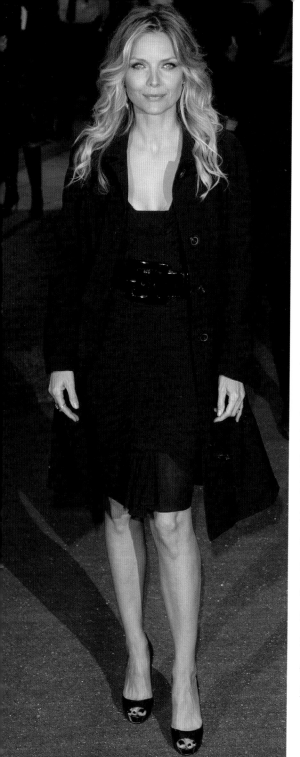

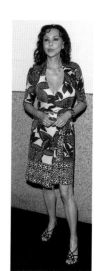

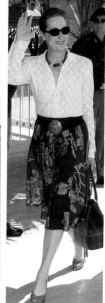

## FIFTIES

Assuming you're happy with your signature styles, update the classics with the new season's colors, fabrics, or fashion elements. If the trend roller coaster is still a thrill ride, by all means shop the look of the moment, but keep an eagle eye out for what works for you. If an entire look doesn't feel right, then sample elements. Of course, after a certain age you'll want to bid farewell to second-skin cling. Jumpsuits, dungarees, cropped tops, rah-rah skirts (or anything similarly twirly) and thigh-high spiky boots go to the charity shop. Even if your body looks great in something, the style has to match your

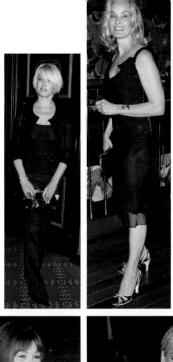

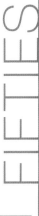

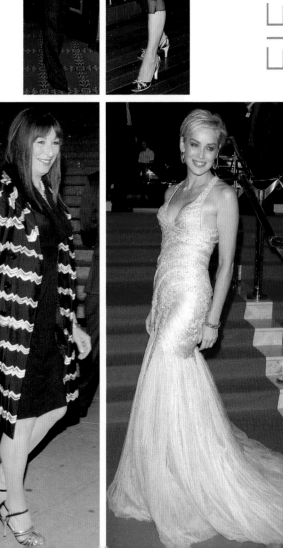

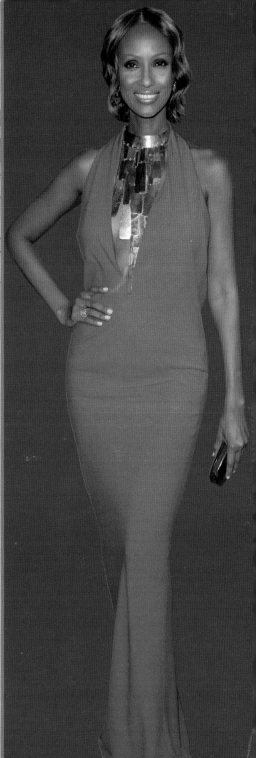

FIFTIES

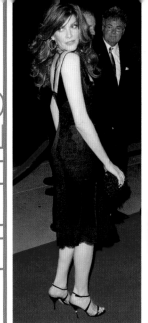

ONE OF MY MOTTOS IS
**FLAUNT WHAT**
　　　　**YOU'VE GOT LEFT.**

Cybill Shepherd

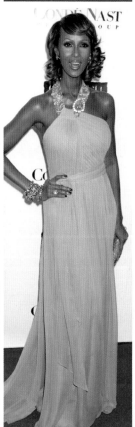

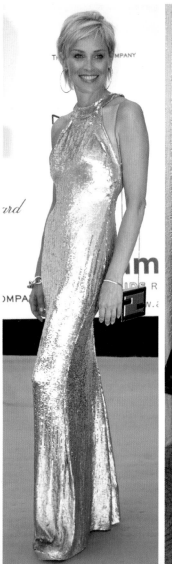

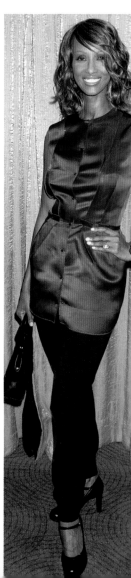

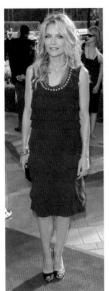
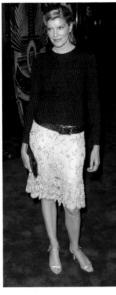
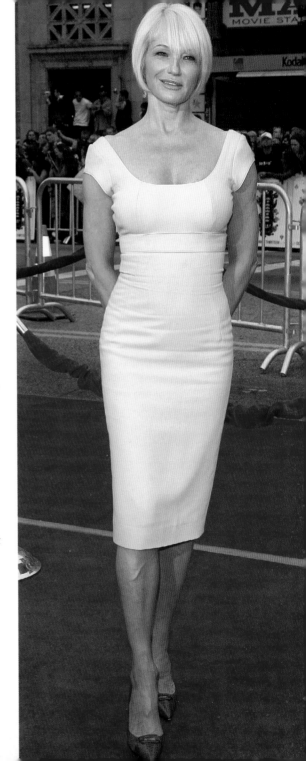

face. But always be wary of that old bugbear "appropriateness." If your skin and figure can take it, there's no reason not to wear low-waist trousers (without baring your midriff) or jean jackets as long as you feel right in them. Feel free to buy the jeans shape of the season, the cool shirt, or hippest handbag. But it's probably enough to let this one key trend be the focus of your look. Tone the rest of it down by keeping everything else simple and basic. Remember that personal style still rules: if you've always been a hippie chick, don't stop now. You just don't need the poncho *and* the turquoise bangles *and* the clogs *and* the caftan *and* the headscarf. Try one of these things at a time.

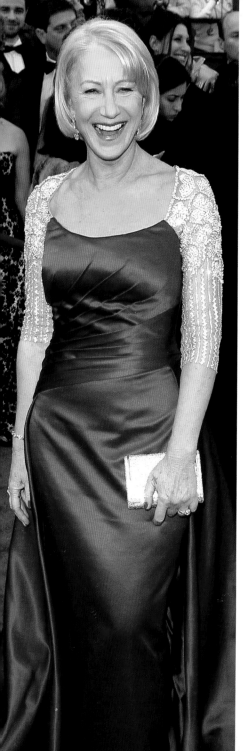

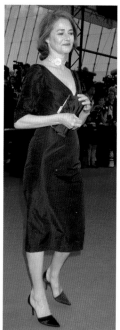
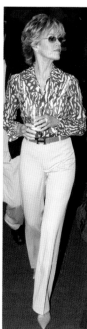

## SIXTIES

Learn to let go of some of the fripperies that some women cling to as they get older. Frills and fussy lines are instantly aging. Clean, simple lines look sharpest. You can carry bold patterns, glamorous metallics, and strong colors. On you they look positively regal. Whimsical details (such as ditsy collars and novelty buttons) or pattern (rose sprigs or country florals) are only for cartoon grandmas. Anything too ladylike after a certain age will look stuffy. Prim suits or matching handbags add instant frump factor.

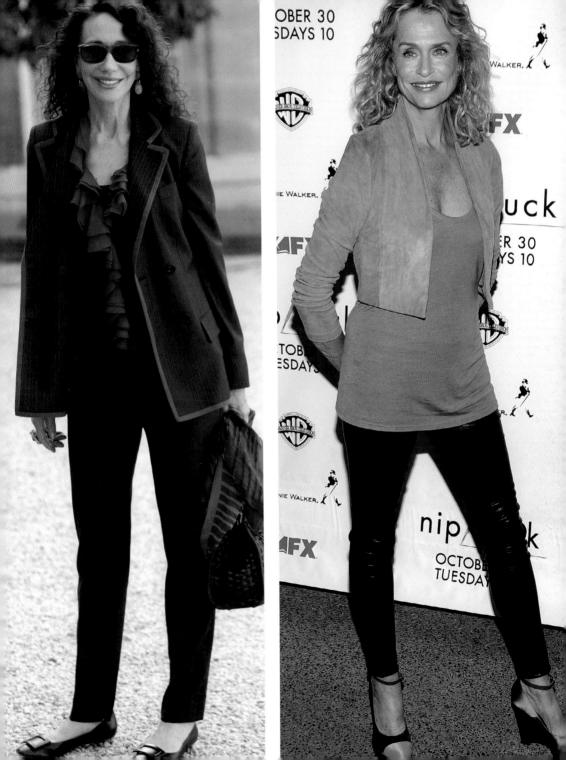

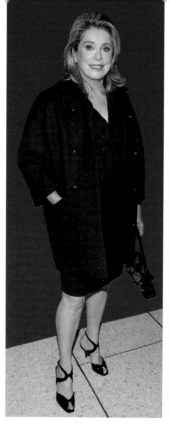
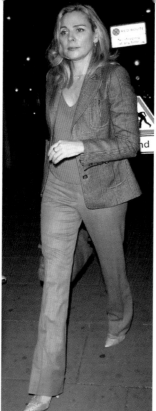
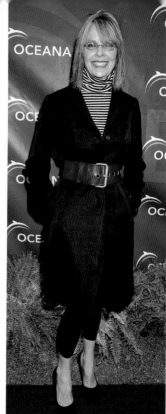

## CAN I HAVE LONG HAIR?

Long hair gives up on us way before we are ready to give up on it. Past the age of forty-five, long hair will have lost some of the lustrous quality that made it look so appealing, flowing down your back at twenty. Now is no time to grow your hair long if you have always worn it short or shoulder length. But if it has always been your look, and you love it, then by all means keep it long. At a certain point, too long hair can be aging. A length that hits just below the shoulder is more flattering. You need to consult with your hairdresser and find a way to balance the elements of control (for the sophisticated, sleek look that you

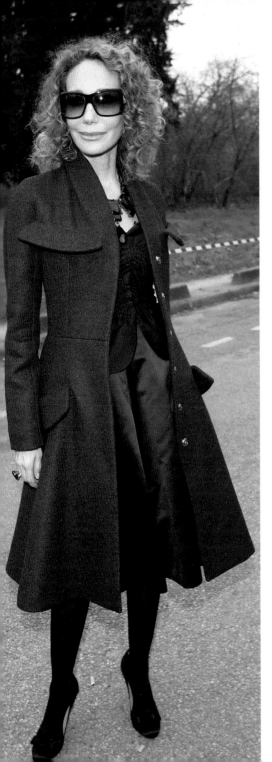

can carry so well) with natural movement. Anything too severely styled is aging, and if your hair is going gray it will make you look like a cartoon granny. Maintenance becomes mandatory—schedule regular trims and conditioning treatments. Long hair in poor condition is not a good look at any age. But long, unkempt hair on any one over forty is instantly aging.

## TO DYE OR NOT TO DYE

A gradual transition to a silken silver gray may be many women's ideal, but it doesn't happen that often; generally it's a more patchy experience. As you mask or blend those grays remember that very dark hair can look harsh with mature skin, so reassess your look with your colorist on a regular basis. If you are dyeing, keep on top of the maintenance. Never let your roots go. Thinking of one last fling with a shock of pink or magenta? Extreme hair on older women looks bad unless, like Patricia Field or Zandra Rhodes, you have built a life around outrageous style statements.

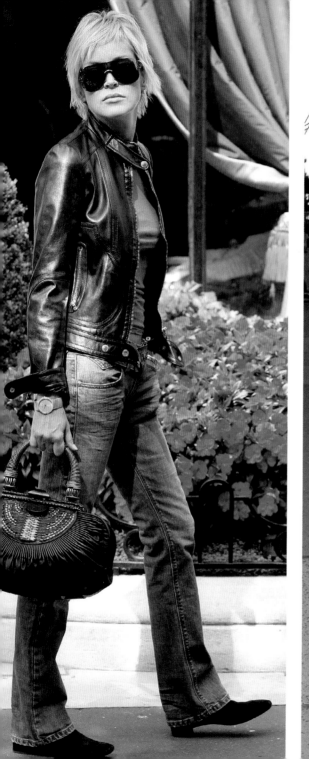
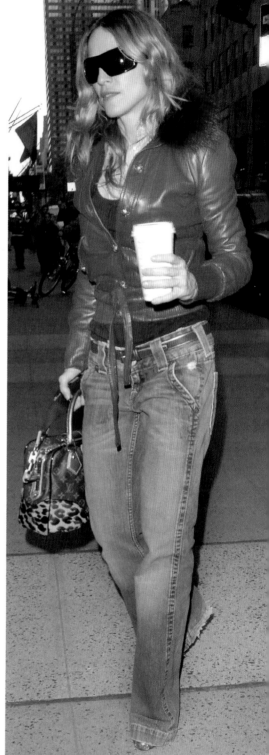

ONLY **ROY ROGERS**
**AND MARLENE DIETRICH**
SHOULD BE ALLOWED
**TO WEAR LEATHER TROUSERS.**

Edith Head

## HOW LONG CAN I KEEP WEARING MY JEANS?

If you love to wear jeans and you have a clear idea of what suits your body shape, then there is no reason not to be wearing them at eighty. As you get older, steer clear of fashion's excesses: bare midriffs, low-slung waistbands that expose body parts conventionally covered by underwear, or extreme flares. Head-to-toe denim can look good on twentysomethings, but after that it makes a stronger statement if you mix it up a little. For example, try your jeans jacket with your simple black skirt or cotton dress.

## WHAT ABOUT LEATHER?

Some women in their forties and beyond look just great in beautifully tailored leather trousers. Others just look like Miss Whiplash's auntie. Unless you are a genuine fifty-year-old biker moll (which means you're actually living the life, not just dressing up as if you do), then a tailored single-breasted leather jacket is bound to look better than what your son thinks is cool to wear when he's burning up the highway. Leather, of beautiful quality in classic shapes, can look sleek and glossy on women of any age. Let leather pieces go the moment they show the shape of your knees, elbows or your bottom when you are not in them.

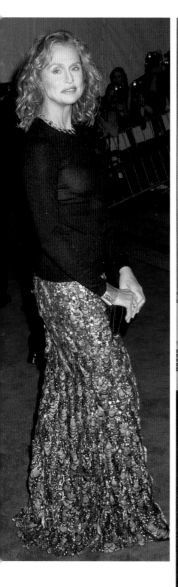

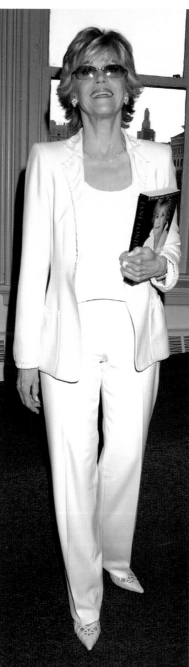

**IT'S ALL RIGHT**
LETTING YOURSELF GO
**AS LONG AS**
YOU CAN GET
YOURSELF BACK.

Mick Jagger

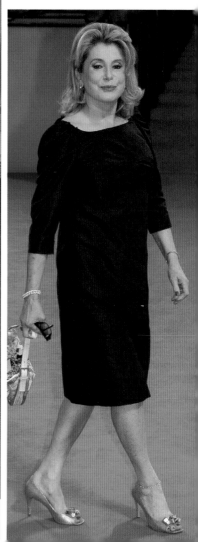

## HOW LOW (OR HIGH) DO YOU GO?

Face it, girls, you've got to have truly stunning legs to do the bare-legged thigh-high mini over thirty-five. If your legs are only so-so, you may duck the deadline for another few years with opaque tights. By forty, your great shape may be surviving middle age, but unless you're one of the genetically gifted (possible, but rare), the tone will have started to go before that. So be scrupulously honest with yourself. A skirt that hits above the knee worn with opaque hose may still cut it. But short shorts, off the beach, are a no-no for anyone over twenty-five. There are sexier erogenous zones in the stylish anatomy: try baring a shoulder, back, or cleavage.

## THE GENERATION TRAP

Young women dressed old beyond their years and older women clinging to the fripperies of youth are both committing mortal style sins.

A sixty-year-old in paint-splash prints, ruffles, or bows or a back-to-front baseball cap is not charming or funny. Likewise, a grandmother with a great body in shapeless tweed is underselling her elegance as badly as a granny in hot pants.

And at the other end of the age scale, the young woman in a boxy suit is as off-putting as her contemporary who's on the way to class dressed as if she's about to make an appearance at the Grammys. And a twenty-year-old in a lumpy cardigan and velvet headband is equally unappealing.

Any kind of pretending is wrong at any age. Being out of touch with what's great about your style is a wasted opportunity at seventeen and a tragedy at seventy. Study what you've got and go with it. Keep pleasure at the front of your mind at all times, and you won't go too far wrong.

6

SECRETS OF THE SUCCESSFUL

S  H  O  P  P  E  R

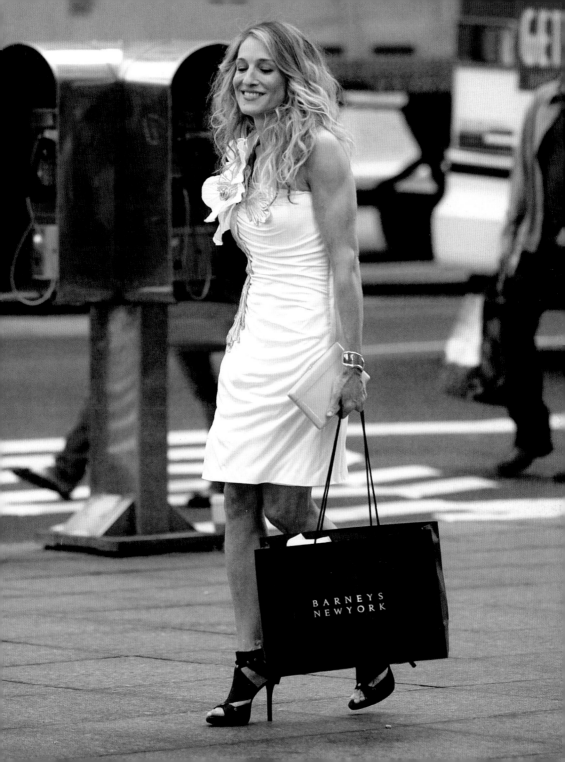

## THERE IS NO DOUBT **A NEW DRESS** **IS A HELP** UNDER ALL CIRCUMSTANCES.

British author Noel Streatfeild

BY NOW YOU SHOULD be starting to have an idea of what looks are emerging from your newly edited wardrobe. You've weeded out the tatty, the old-fashioned, the worn out, the stretched, and the just plain wrong stuff. If looking at your dwindling collection is giving you separation anxiety, console yourself: it's honestly better to do without than make do with something you know is wrong. If it makes you look dumpy, frumpy, or ordinary, it does not deserve wardrobe space.

The clothes you're left with should be:

- Those that make you look good. You can throw them on even if you have only minutes to get ready and, for the time you are wearing them, just know you have nothing more to worry about on that score. Great style is stress-free!

- Those that are comfortable. Suffering for the sake of fashion was the mantra of a man with sales commission on his mind. True, you can't wear your PJs to a dressy party and there are times when, for a fabulous shoe, you will be prepared to pay a physical price. But remember, nothing is more luxurious than comfort. No one looks chicer than a woman at ease. You can't look good if you don't feel good. Sure, make a sacrifice, but draw the line at being a victim and resolve never again to be too cold, in pain, asphyxiated by your waistband, *or* stuck in a muddy field with spiky high heels on.

Assemble these clothes into outfits and work out what you need to really finish them off (could be a belt, a new white T-shirt, or a fine-

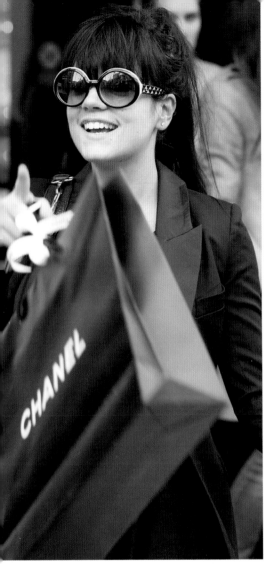

## SOME USEFUL LISTS

First, the *Basics* (everyday knits, jeans, casual pants, and T-shirts). Because you wear them a lot, there will be a relatively high turnover in these items to keep them fresh and up-to-date. *Tailored items* will betray your budget, so be careful. Better to have one great pair of tailored trousers that upgrades every outfit you build around them than several pairs of shoddy quality that drag your look down. If the pair that makes you look best will break the bank account, wait for the sales, scour the outlets, or check the Internet for a better deal. Don't give up without a fight. *Disposables*, such as T-shirts and cotton shirts, look better box-fresh, so don't break the bank here.

Second, the *Essentials* (a great coat, a fitted suit, a stunning dress, almost all shoes). These items define your silhouette and your style. Buy the best you can afford. Look after them carefully. Plan to get at least a couple of seasons' wear from them.

gauge sweater in a color you don't normally buy). A list focuses every shopping trip. Write down what you need and keep it with you at all times so that you're prepared, even if the unexpected opportunity presents itself.

**WHEN I SEE PEOPLE** DRESSED IN
HIDEOUS CLOTHES **THAT LOOK ALL WRONG ON THEM,**
I TRY TO IMAGINE THE MOMENT
**WHEN THEY WERE BUYING THEM AND THOUGHT,**
"THIS IS GREAT. I LIKE IT. I'LL TAKE IT."

Andy Warhol

The rest, *Trends*—pure eye candy: your nod to passing fads. Make free with your fashion inspiration here, but be wary of anything that looks like the national dress of another country or something you wore ten years ago! Hot trends have built-in obsolescence, the fashion equivalent of fast food. They can come from markets, secondhand shops, and the mall. Buy them, love them, wear them, and, when their fashion nanomoment has passed, dump them.

Successful shoppers think of each new purchase as an extension of what they already have. They hone in on seasonless fabrics (cotton, lightweight wool, silk, jerseys, and fine knits) and clothes with simple lines that can be layered or work just as well alone.

## WHAT YOU NEED TO KNOW BEFORE YOU SPEND

### YOUR LIFESTYLE

- Who are you trying to be (perfect mother, CEO, Oscar winner)?
- Do you have to attend lots of meetings?
- Do you socialize a lot for work, or in order to support your partner?
- Do you commute, walk, or cycle to work every day or work from home? (If you work from home, do you need five business suits? If you work in an office, you may not need another pair of jeans and sneakers.)

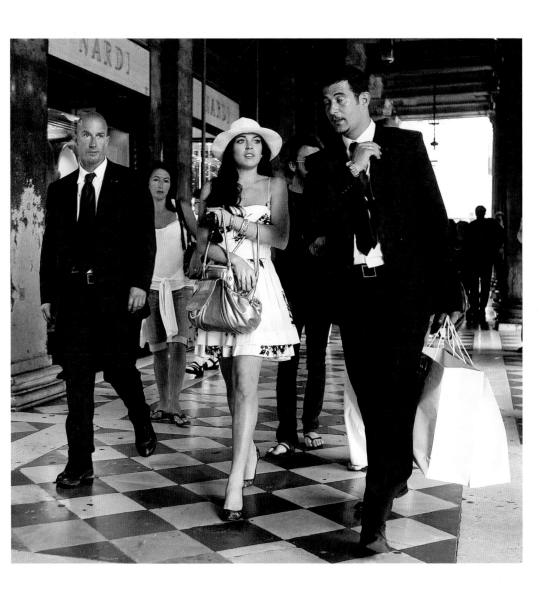

I KEPT IN TOUCH **WITH THE NEEDS** OF WOMEN
WHO HAD **CONFIDENCE IN ME AND**
TRIED TO HELP THEM FIND THEIR TYPE.
THIS I BELIEVED **TO BE THE SECRET OF**
**BEING WELL DRESSED.**

Elsa Schiaparelli

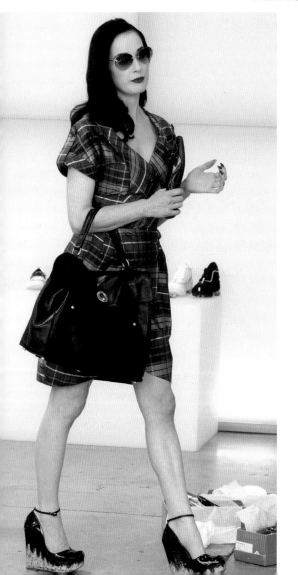

## YOUR BODY

- Are you pear-shaped, round, petite, tall?
- Are your shoulders wide or narrow?
- Do you have a large or small bust?
- Are you short- or long-waisted?
  (See page 75.)

Be honest. Get a sense of what your body
is really like. You simply cannot dress like
Jennifer Lopez if you have a body like
Calista Flockhart.

## WHAT MAKES YOU HAPPY?

- What color do you love that makes you
  feel great?
- What trouser/dress/skirt/jacket shape do
  you feel most comfortable in?
- What's your favorite fabric?

It could be that you have already spotted a common denominator. There is nothing wrong with building your wardrobe on this. It's the firmest foundation you'll ever get. If you love shift dresses, have daytime shift dresses, evening shift dresses, weekend shift dresses. Some may be long, others short. Some may be conservative, others more revealing. If you're addicted to slim pants, go for them every chance you get. In spring, show a little more leg with a shorter crop. In winter, go for an ankle length and more subdued fabrics. Your style reflects different looks but essentially, they're all your favorite pants.

Things like these make up your style signature. You can adapt it, but don't ever change it.

One more thing: stylish women are all different. They are tall, short, classic, eccentric, rich, broke, long-legged, big-boobed, gray-haired, blond, or simply have something you can't quite put your finger on—an elegance that just radiates from within. But, ever since fashion became a seasonal circus, the only thing they have all had in common is the discipline to "just say no" to some of the worst fashion mistakes their decades could tempt them with.

As you become sure of your personal style, you'll buy fewer but better clothes. You'll look great, have more wardrobe space, and be able to pack without freaking out. For each person, it's a constant process of trial and error. Gradually, you'll understand what works for you and makes you feel comfortable and look great. You'll know what to buy immediately and what to leave to your sisters with longer/shorter legs, wider/narrower hips, fuller/flatter chests (no matter what a "bargain" it is).

**YOU HAVE TO** LOOK AT YOURSELF OBJECTIVELY. **ANALYZE YOURSELF** LIKE AN INSTRUMENT. **YOU HAVE TO BE ABSOLUTELY FRANK.** FACE YOUR HANDICAPS, DON'T TRY TO HIDE THEM. **INSTEAD, DEVELOP SOMETHING ELSE.**

Audrey Hepburn

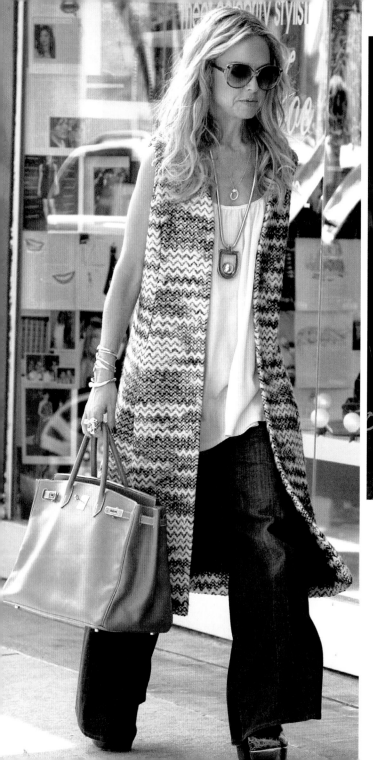

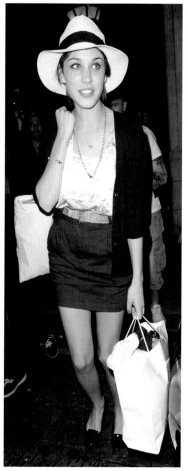

I LIKE TO WALK DOWN **BOND STREET** **THINKING OF** ALL THE THINGS **I DON'T WANT.**

Essayist and critic Logan Pearsall Smi

**TREND AVOIDANCE FEELS LIKE** ASSERTIVENESS IN THE FACE OF **A DOWNPOUR OF INDISCRIMINATE FASHION:** THE RACKS UPON RACKS **THAT SAY** **"BE PART OF THIS," LULLING YOU INTO** **FASHION'S** WOMAN-TRAP— BELONGING.

British journalist Bethan Cole

## THE A TO Z OF A SAVVY SHOPPER

**ALONE** You stand a better chance if you spend a day without having to handle other people's impressions of you. You can go at your own pace and cover old ground repeatedly, and there'll be no one there to question your unbeatable bargain.

**BROWSE** Go slowly and don't be overly ambitious. You probably won't be able to afford your wish list in one go, but even if you could, you probably wouldn't have time and, even if you did, you probably couldn't

find everything at once. So decide which three or four pieces you need most, plus two secondary items. Write these down, too. Don't forget to keep upcoming weddings, parties, and other important occasions in mind.

**BUDGET** Set one . . . not for each piece, but for each shopping day. Be flexible and open to surprises, but think of your mortgage once you hit your limit. If you know you can't stop yourself, get your day's budget from the cash machine and leave your credit card at home. If you have to break it (for the coat, boots, suit you have always dreamt of—not the sequined jumpsuit

**I'M THE SORT OF PERSON WHO CUTS THE LABEL ON THINGS.** I HATE THE WHOLE IDEA OF A SEASONAL MUST-HAVE. I THINK **CLOTHING THAT SCREAMS ITS ORIGINS** TO PEOPLE IN THE STREET **IS UNCOMFORTABLE** IN A WORLD WHERE **LOTS OF PEOPLE DON'T HAVE LOTS OF MONEY.**

Thomas Maier, designer of Bottega Veneta

in the shop window) and you know your budget is nonnegotiable, be prepared to drop something else from your shopping list. Make sure that what you like complements your existing wardrobe. If it doesn't go with what you have, you could be creating a need for more stuff (and more spending).

**CBS** A fabulous Coat, Bag, and Shoes are the most direct route to looking great. There's a tribe of extremely stylish women out there who put their faith in the power of this simple formula. These items are what people see first. Get them right and what's underneath can be as simple and as basic as you like.

**COLOR** When deciding how to build your perfect wardrobe, focusing on a color can be a good start. Black is an obvious basic. But be honest—is it draining your skin? It's so unkind to most pale northern European skins, particularly in winter. Try dark navy blue or dark gray instead.

**DEPRESSION** If you shop when you're feeling low you are bound to make mistakes. See a good movie instead.

**ENOUGH** One or two slip dresses are fine for the summer, but a whole wardrobe full is too much like hard work.

**ESSENTIALS** Buy them at the beginning of the season, when you have the most choice. Leave fashion indulgences for the sales.

**EVENINGWEAR** The night can transform a flea market dress into a stunning statement. But unless the quality is impeccable, secondhand can look second-rate at the office. Working women need to spend more money on daywear than eveningwear. For you, daytime is when looking like you have it together pays dividends.

**FADS** Just because pink is in fashion doesn't mean it should be in your wardrobe. Fads and trends come and go. Use fashion to develop and enhance your style, not as an excuse to abandon it altogether. Stick to your guns. If red is your color, it works no

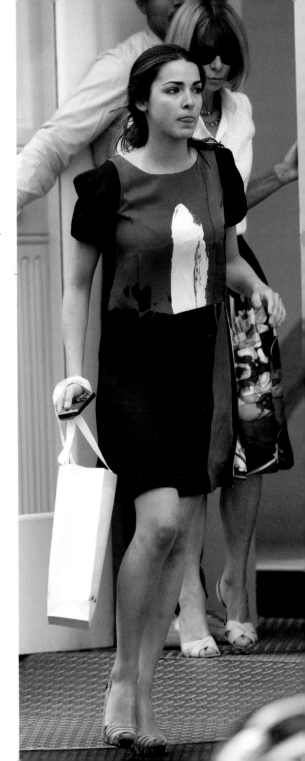

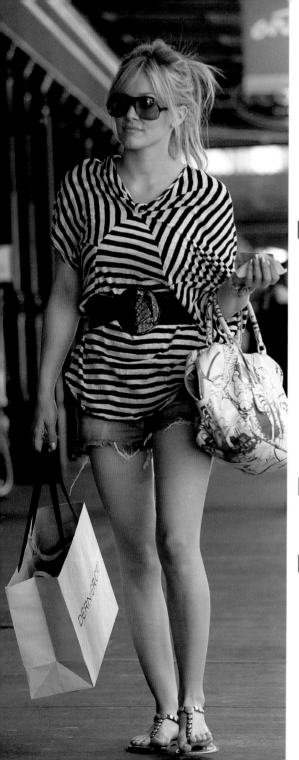

matter what the current hot fashion shade. If cropped trousers make you look stumpy, avoid them, no matter how trendy they are. Looking good is about self-awareness, not what others say is hip.

**FOUNDATION** Never stop trying to get this just right. Certain pieces will be the cornerstone of your wardrobe. They may not be expensive, or have designer labels, or even be the newest items in your wardrobe, but they're the key pieces that will help you get to work on time knowing that you look great, and without wasting precious time trying to match weird colors.

**GREED** If you really love something and you know it works for you, buy two.

**HOMEWORK** If you do it right, before you shop, you'll get the biggest bang for your buck! Keep clippings from magazines of looks you love. As you do this, a clearer picture will start to emerge of what ought to be in your essentials list. Be honest with yourself. If you would never wear a miniskirt, skip those pictures of leggy models in microminis. If one particular item keeps recurring (slim black skirt, trench coat), it can feature high on your list of priorities.

**INTERNET SHOPPING** Oh, the joy of an evening in bed with a laptop, shopping your favorite site. One of my favorite pastimes is to fill my basket with items for my ideal wardrobe and then never check out. Hours of harmless fun can be had this way and in the process, valuable style insight and confidence gained as you stretch your virtual style sense. If you are not ready to commit, leave your favorites on your wish list and give yourself some thinking time. You are more likely to be able to identify your personal essentials if you allow some time for the fever of your fantasy shopping spree to pass. And getting e-mail alerts about the new stuff that's just arrived is way more fun than a mall trawl.

**JUNK** Toss anything that challenges your shape instead of flattering it. Also in this category are cheap fabrics that need steam and dry cleaning to make them look good. They're not at all cheap—they're expensive junk masquerading as a bargain.

**KNOWLEDGE** Know when your favorite store has its seasonal sales. Know the best secondhand shops, the best stalls at flea markets, the best sites on the Internet. Know where the outlet shops are (not just at home, but near where you may be on vacation, too). Keep an eagle eye on the papers for designer warehouse sales. There are ways you need never pay full price for anything, but this requires some serious attention.

**LAST-MINUTE** Shopping right before an event invariably leads to overspending on something you don't like much.

**MEMORY** Not to be trusted. If you're looking for a piece to wear with another, bring the item you need a match for.

**NETWORK** Develop relationships with staff in shops you like. You'll get much better service this way. Call ahead and check if they have what you want. Ask for the shop assistant by name. Introduce yourself when you get to the shop. Write his/her name down and remember it. If they know you and what you want, they'll call you next time it comes in. If your local department store has a personal shopping service, try it out. Good personal shoppers are an invaluable resource, and you don't have to spend a fortune to use one. Don't forget, time-strapped shoppers can also access personal shopping services through online retailers.

**OBVIOUS** Conspicuous display of designer logos is just not cool.

**PATIENCE** Accept that it takes time to get good at this.

**PREPARATION** The shopping process is way easier if you wear lightweight garments that can be slipped on and off. Straight skirts and V-necked sweaters, opaque hose, and flat slip-on shoes are all good. If you go shopping in tricky outfits, you're almost guaranteed to be in a bad mood after two trips to the fitting room. Do your hair and makeup, so you don't look awful in everything. Dress to shop—you'll feel better and you'll get better service.

**QUESTION** Constantly ask yourself: Does it fit? Does it go with what I already have? Does it work for or against me?

**RESEARCH** Decide where you're going before you set out. The source information from your clippings may help you work this out. Wandering aimlessly around the mall is a demoralizing experience unless you happen to come across the thing you love by chance—a rare occurrence.

**SALES** Be wary of getting carried away. Don't buy something on sale you wouldn't

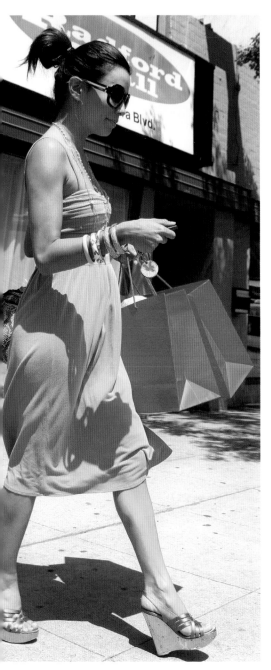

pay full price for—it's not a bargain if it isn't great. Avoid buying stuff you don't need. You can go wrong with something that costs $20. Once it's in your wardrobe, the price tags are off. It's what fits and looks good that matters. Bear in mind that it's not always wise to wait for a sale, because anything you really want may very well be gone by then.

**SPLURGE** The key to success here is to know when. Don't spend weeks hunting for something slightly better or cheaper. If you love it, get it.

**SYNDROMES** "Spending the rent on red shoes" is the one your mother warned you about. Fashion mistakes aren't just those that make your skin look sallow or your stomach fat. They can be fabulous things for which you need not another body, but another life.

**TAILOR** A reliable one should be every woman's key contact. The secret to making inexpensive clothes look good is a great tailor.

But not every seam can be tampered with. If a jacket doesn't fit right in the shoulders or lie flat when buttoned, get over it. Don't buy anything that's badly finished. If a garment needs shortening or needs the waist nipped in, fine. But if it needs more, forget it. Mutant tailoring looks terrible on anybody.

**UNDERWEAR** Well-fitted lingerie will make you look better in clothes. Wear a flesh-toned, seamless bra. Use control-top hose to smooth your silhouette. If you're trying on trousers, wear a thong or high-waisted panties.

**VENTURE OUT** Visit designer shops even if you think they're beyond your budget. You'll get ideas. And if you try on expensive, well-made clothes, you'll get a sense of what a great cut feels like. If you're well-organized, it's possible to build an entire look with budget items bought around a key designer piece. Be daring and try on things that you might not think are "you." You may be

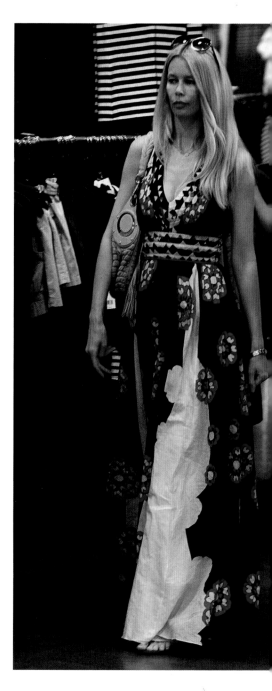

pleasantly surprised. Don't ignore something just because it has no hanger appeal. It could look great on your body.

**VERSATILITY** If you can't see yourself in more than five completely different situations in an item, don't buy it (unless it's sportswear, eveningwear, or a wedding dress).

**WEIGHT** Don't buy anything you need to slim down to fit into (especially anything from your essentials list). Unless it's a bathing suit, most garments fit best a bit loose. A skimming fit will make you look thinner. A tight fit will create an illusion of extra poundage.

**X FACTOR** Be nice to yourself. If you're hopelessly in love with something, don't let your fashion demons nag you with "What do you need it for, and where will you wear it?" You may not need it or have anywhere to wear it right now, but imagine the fun you'll have when you do.

**YEARNING** If you're in doubt as to whether something is really worth a splurge, leave it. If you can't tough it out, ask them to hold it. If you still love it the next day, chances are it's a good buy. If you're over it, you'll be relieved you can invest somewhere else.

**ZEALOT** Fashion is fun, not a religion. Identify the trend and adapt your favorites to show you are fashion savvy but not a fashion victim.

I DON'T **REALLY** HAVE A SECRET. I JUST TRY TO WEAR **MATCHING** COLORS.

Ben Stiller

# 7

## HOW TO CHOOSE A

## COAT

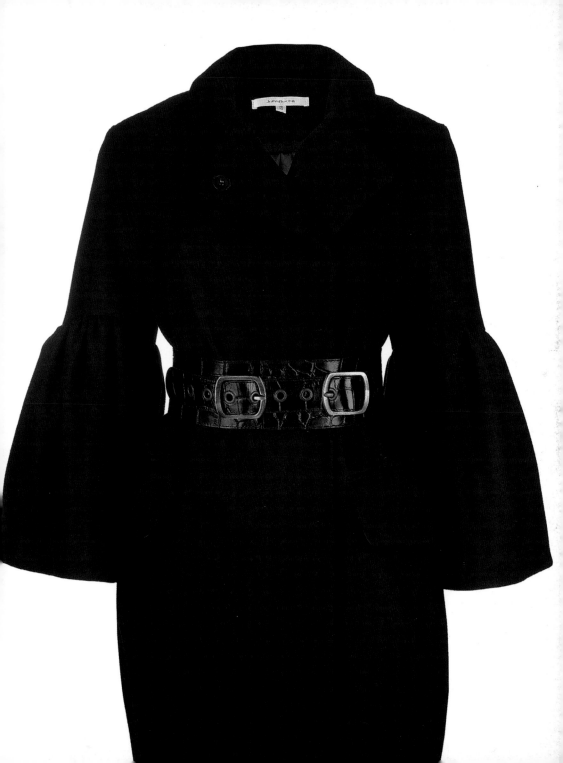

THIS MORNING **CAME HOME MY FINE CLOAK,**
WITH GOLD BUTTON . . . **WHICH COST ME
MUCH MONEY,** AND I PRAY GOD TO MAKE ME ABLE
**TO PAY FOR IT.**

British parliamentarian and diarist Samuel Pepys

A GREAT COAT MAKES serious style impact. Like a fabulous handbag or chic shoe, it can pull your look together in a moment. It can express your mood or style like nothing else. And, even if everything underneath is less than perfect, that coat will add polish in an instant. Use it to make an entrance. Use it to camouflage figure faults. Use it to make your style statement. The right coat makes everything look better. Buy the best you can afford, and the style payback will astonish you.

## THE PERFECT COAT
## CAPSULE WARDROBE

A great coat must deliver not just on style but on warmth, longevity, and versatility. It makes more first impressions than any other item in your wardrobe. It's a major purchase, so take some time to work out your strategy before you shop.

- There's no such thing as the perfect coat. No one garment will work as well for the office as it does for the evening, the weekend, or in driving rain. Of course, you may find one coat that does double duty, but avoid setting yourself up for disappointment and frustration by thinking you'll be able to find one style that suits all occasions.

- The complete coat wardrobe goes something like this:

1. One coat for day that is roughly knee length (depending on your height and body type)

2. An evening coat

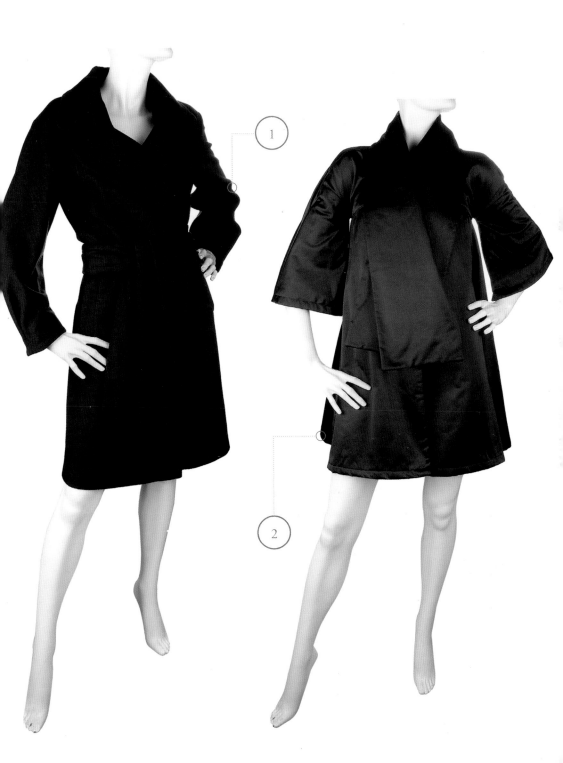

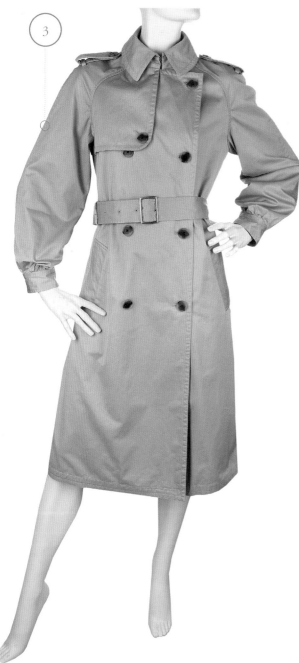

(3)

3. A raincoat

4. A cold-weather parka (if your local weather calls for it)

5. Something laid-back for the weekend

When considering your priorities, three of these five are key: you could double up on the day and evening coats if you find one that can make the transition with style; your weekend and cold-weather needs could be answered by one. Money spent on a trench coat will never be regretted. It is the chicest, most useful, and most versatile coat ever invented.

- When it comes to how your coat is made, be picky. Do not compromise on quality. Coats are one of the best investments you can make in your own style.

- The simpler the coat, the more versatile and the longer it will last looking good. Extra-wide lapels, shiny buttons, wide shoulders, and crazy colors make statements, but they also limit the life of your coat.

- Think about your daily routine: How much of your day is spent sitting in cars

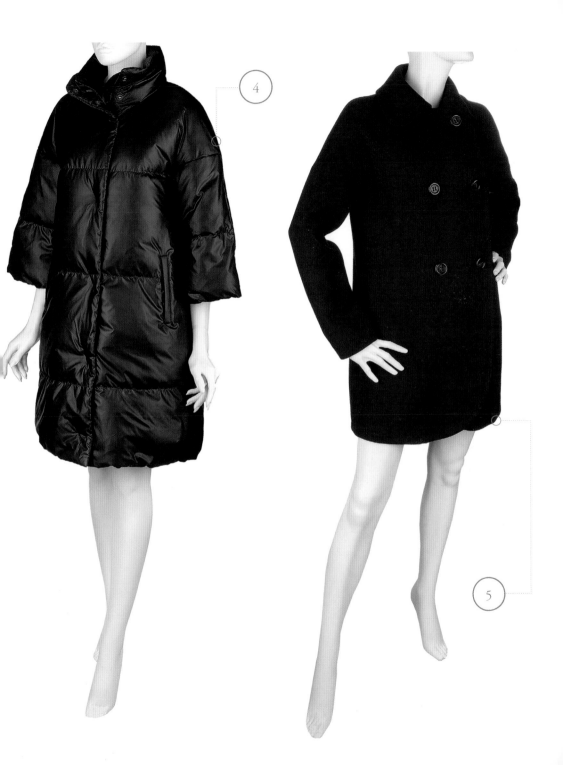

4

5

or other vehicles? Someone who walks to work may need a knee-length sheepskin, but you don't want a big coat dragging up the steps of the bus or tangled around you in the car. And you don't want a bulky coat if you often have to stand up in a crush of humanity on the bus or train. How much time do you spend outside and exposed to the elements? How often will your coat be bundled up inside an aircraft's overhead bin, and how often will it be worn under a baby carrier?

- Think about what you'll be wearing under your coat. If you wear a lot of jackets, try the coat on with a jacket underneath. If you wear mostly lighter pieces, be sure the coat is snug enough so it doesn't overwhelm you. Consider your favorite skirt lengths. Old rules dictated that your coat should cover your hemline, but as with most hard-and-fast fashion rules these days, that no longer applies. Practically speaking, it's a good idea to have your coat hem longer than your skirt to keep it dry. But then trench coats look pretty good with an inch or two of skirt showing. Mid-thigh–length coats look cute with a slightly longer skirt underneath, and a successful boho look often depends on having a bit of skirt showing. If you are going for a look that is sleek and polished, buy your coat slightly longer than your skirts.

- Consider the climate where you live and work: Arctic chill? Wet? Or is it unpredictable, making layers under a lighter coat more practical? Sheepskin is a great insulator against cold and wind, but terrible in wet weather. Lined leather is great for windy places, but a synthetic is better for rainier climates.

- Is this purchase for fun or investment? If you want it to last for years, then go for the most classic shape and neutral color.

- What colors are in your wardrobe? If you wear neutrals, then a coat in a bright color like red or orange is a better buy than you think. It will complement, not clash, with your outfits and add a whole new dimension to your look.

- Be adventurous. A great coat in an unexpected color, fabric, or shape can be just as versatile as the standard classics and will give even the simplest wardrobe a shot of chic.

- Bright coats in classic shapes easily do weekend and work duty, but you'll maximize their versatility if you stick to matte fabrics (wool, flannel, cashmere).

## FIGURE WARNINGS

- The most versatile coat for almost all figures is a narrow, figure-skimming, three-quarter length coat (hits right on or below the knee). It is both modern and flattering. Curvier figures look good in its figure-skimming sleekness. If you are big-bosomed, go for an open collar that is cut on the wide side. It will never look dated.

- A soft, belted style is the next most versatile shape for most figures. It works

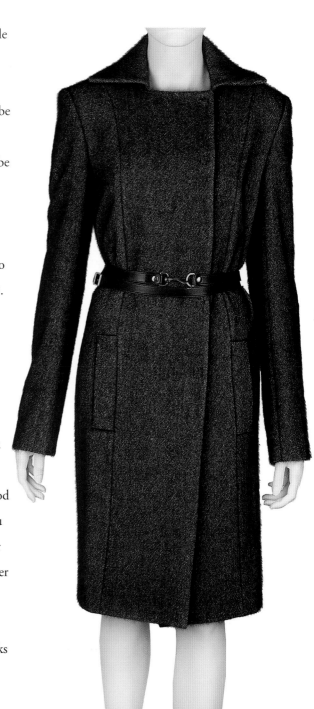

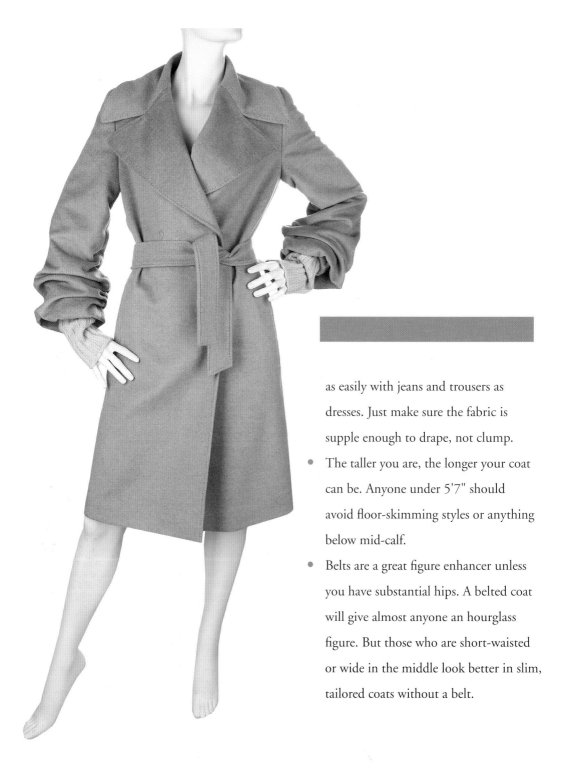

as easily with jeans and trousers as dresses. Just make sure the fabric is supple enough to drape, not clump.

- The taller you are, the longer your coat can be. Anyone under 5'7" should avoid floor-skimming styles or anything below mid-calf.

- Belts are a great figure enhancer unless you have substantial hips. A belted coat will give almost anyone an hourglass figure. But those who are short-waisted or wide in the middle look better in slim, tailored coats without a belt.

- If you are curvy, accentuating the narrowest part of your body—your waist—will give instant glamour. Belted coats, whether they hit below the knee or mid-thigh, look good. But a three-quarter length coat that skims the body will look even better. Short, boxy styles will make your curves look bulky. So will voluminous A-lines that drop from the shoulders. Stick to tailored, curve-friendly options.

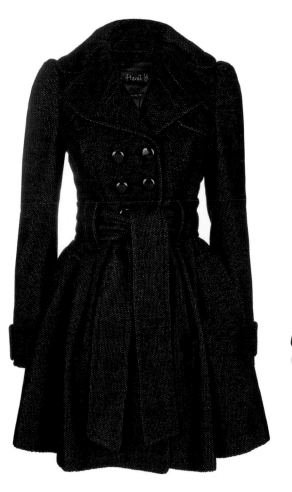

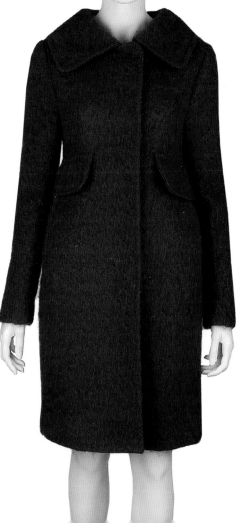

- Puffy parkas only work on slim women. If you don't want to add extra poundage, opt for unpadded versions.

- If you're going for a clean silhouette, be wary of thick, bulky fabrics. They will compromise the sleekness you are aiming for.

- On petite women, belted shapes that sit on or just above the knee will look great. Short coats will increase leg length.

- Proportion is the most important thing in a coat that flatters. You must take time to assess how the bulk of a coat affects your figure. It can do good things (such as smoothing over problem areas) as easily as bad (adding width where you don't need it). So try to be as objective as possible.

- There's no easier way to update your basic look than to slip on a coat with a little attitude: op-art patterns, vintage, printed leather.

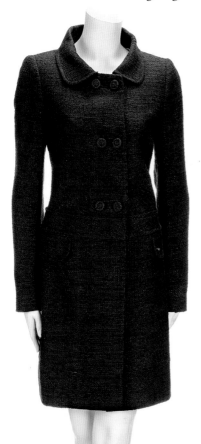
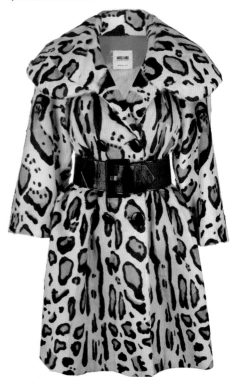

# A PERFECT COAT
# FOR EVERY OCCASION

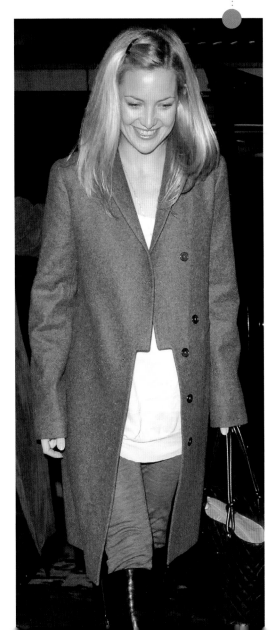

EVERYDAY COAT

- Don't get caught up in the hottest trends. This one will be expected to last. A simple cut in a basic color will see you through several seasons. (But note that basic does not always mean black or beige—if a bright color works with your day-to-day wardrobe and feels right, go for it.)

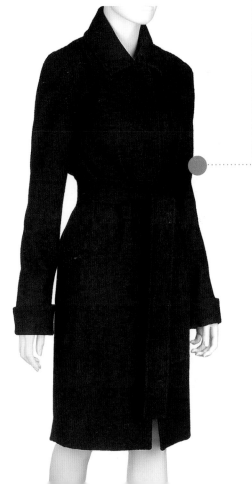

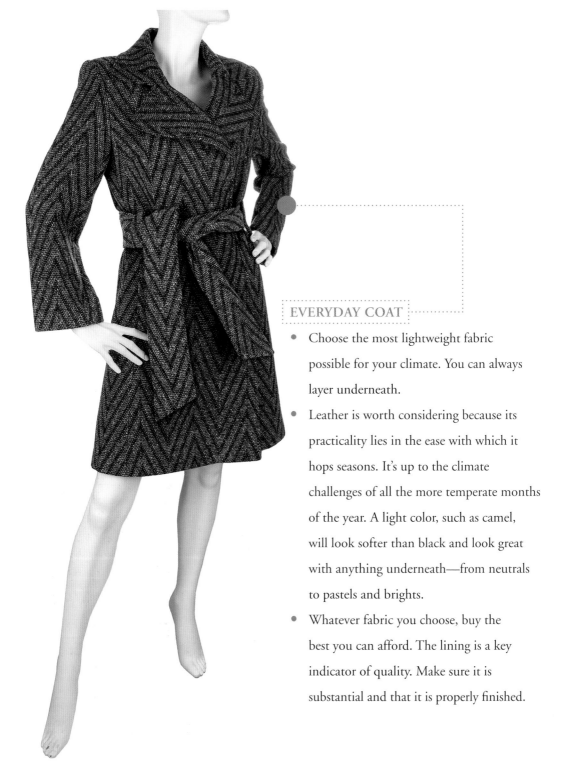

## EVERYDAY COAT

- Choose the most lightweight fabric possible for your climate. You can always layer underneath.

- Leather is worth considering because its practicality lies in the ease with which it hops seasons. It's up to the climate challenges of all the more temperate months of the year. A light color, such as camel, will look softer than black and look great with anything underneath—from neutrals to pastels and brights.

- Whatever fabric you choose, buy the best you can afford. The lining is a key indicator of quality. Make sure it is substantial and that it is properly finished.

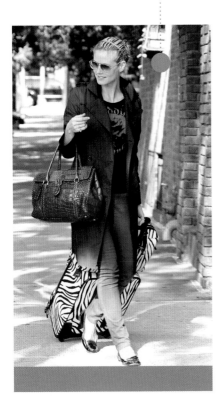

- Lightweight is the key here. Double-faced wool (two layers of wool woven together) or cashmere (the ultimate luxury) are perfect. Because the fabric is double-sided, they don't need a lining and can be rolled and packed without creasing. Because they look so sleek and sharp, they can often sub for a jacket if worn open over basic layers underneath.

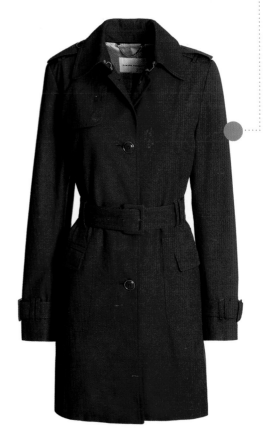

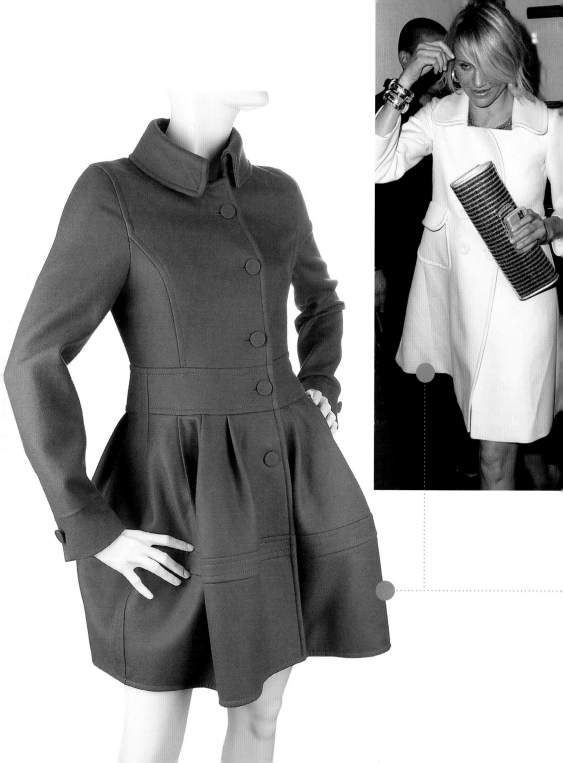

- This will probably not be the first coat you buy, but if you can afford a second, it will add great polish to jeans and tailored pieces and finish off cocktail dresses. Keep shapes simple—high armholes, few pockets, small collars—and let the drama come from the detail: fabric, pattern, embroidery, print, texture.

- Limit fur to trim . . . any more and you're moving into an evening look.

- If you're going for an all-over pattern, choose one with a neutral background for the most mileage.

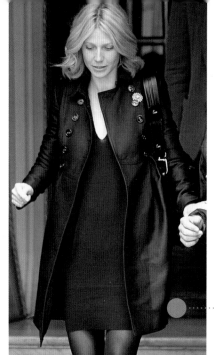

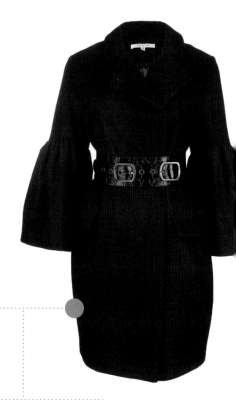

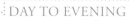

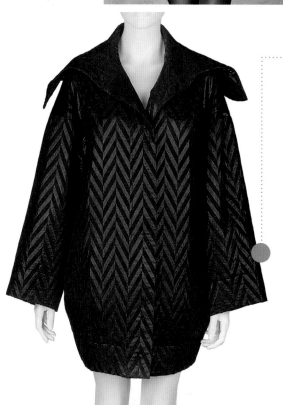

DAY TO EVENING

- To slip seamlessly from work into a night out, look for a simply cut coat in a neutral color. Really consider the length—three-quarters is safe, and it works with most dresses.

- Go for fabrics with sheen or texture (glossy wools, subtle brocades). A classic shape in an unexpected fabric can go dressy, but be grounded enough for day or weekend wear (such as a patent trench or white peacoat).

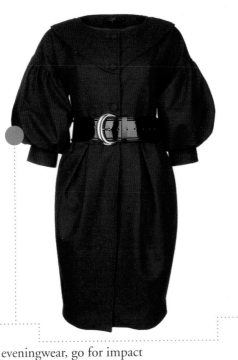

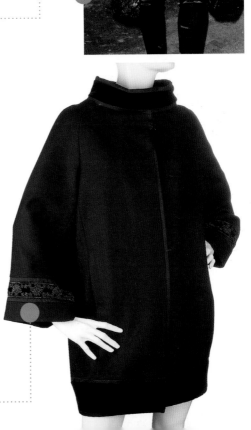

## EVENING

- For dressy eveningwear, go for impact in a simple, well-cut coat with just a hint of detailing. A luxurious fur collar, especially one in a contrasting color, will add drama. For something more subdued, go with a straightforward silhouette in an interesting fabric with some sheen or texture. Velvets, satins, brocades, and silks are perfect.

- Off-white for evening is a great alternative to the blacks and grays. Because it is unexpected, it always turns heads. It goes with everything and adds light to your face and complexion.

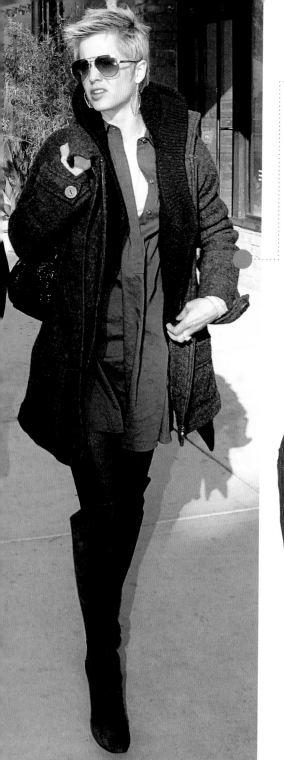

- The sporty cousin to your serious work overcoat, a casual coat can and should express your personality. A peacoat or three-quarter length leather is sophisticated, while a bright, quilted parka or duffle coat has a youthful attitude.

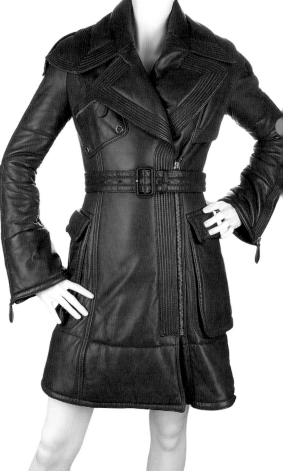

## THE TRENCH

This is an essential wardrobe item. It travels well, is inherently chic, covers a multitude of sins, creates a sharp first impression, goes with jeans and cocktail dresses, beats the windiest and wettest weather, and . . . it *never* goes out of style.

The trench looks as good at night as during the day. It's a basic principle of Parisian chic that a trench coat slung over your cocktail dress has an irresistible charm.

- You can wear it long, short, new, secondhand, crumpled, or crisp, but not dirty.

- You can buckle or tie your belt, but don't cinch your trench too tightly or it will bunch around the waist.

- Don't tie your buckle at the back. It looks tacky.

- Small women look good in trenches if they keep the details simple: big epaulettes, voluminous cuts, and wide lapels are out. Choose a length cut above the knee or shorter.

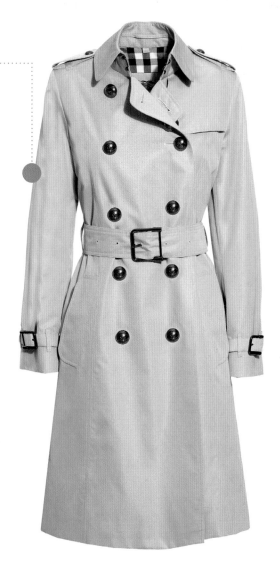

- Single-breasted coats are generally the most flattering. The extra rows of buttons on double-breasted coats can create an illusion of width.

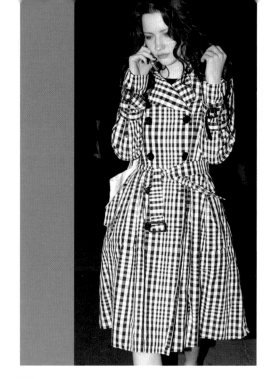

### Anatomy of the Trench

- Cut: Keep it slim. Too much of such an intricately detailed garment will add weight. It's not your goal to look like a big beige bird, flapping down the street.

- Epaulettes: Be sure those shoulders are not sloppy and that they neatly follow your natural shoulder line.

- Storm flap: Not just a fashion detail. This is purposely designed to give you extra protection and insulation about the shoulders.

- Belt: A classic trench needs a belt. If it doesn't have one, it's just a mac. A leather-bound buckle will not last as long as a resin or metal one: after a few good tugs you may begin to find bald patches.

- Fantail pleat: A well-cut trench should have an inverted pleat at the center back for ease of movement.

- Cuff straps: They ought to be adjustable to help seal off inner sleeves from wintry drafts.

### Fabric

- The classic trench is made from cotton gabardine—a fabric with an extremely tight weave that is then treated to make it waterproof. But this is no longer the only option: matte silk, matte stretch, microfiber, or nylon also work.

- If you are looking for wrinkle resistance, avoid lightweight cotton fabrics. Cotton or polyester blends are better.

- A leather trench makes a sharp statement but suffers in the rain, so steer clear if it's your first buy.

## THE PARKA

This jacket is a workhorse. It's meant to keep you warm and dry in the dead of winter. But let's not forget that looking cool is half the equation here.

### The Look

- Thigh length is practical. Longer hinders mobility, and shorter means your bottom is not protected.

- The most flattering looks are nipped in at the waist rather than boxy.

- Military neutrals (khaki or buff), black, and white are the most versatile colors.

- If you feel it, go glamorous, and wear it over an evening gown or tuxedo suit in the evening. It looks great.

### Parka Lowdown

- Fill: A jacket's warmth is determined mainly by its filling or lining.

- Down fill: Warm, lightweight, and compressible, down is the most fantastic insulator. A coat can contain up to 30 percent feathers (not as warm as down—feel for the quills) and still be called

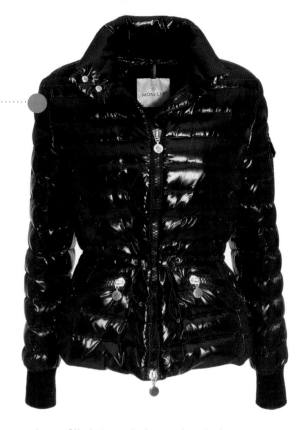

down-filled. Down's downside: It's slow to dry.

- Synthetic fill: Good-quality synthetics such as polyester microfiber feel almost like down and can be just as warm. They are also faster-drying and amazingly compressible. Look for names such as Polarguard, PrimaLoft, and Microtemp.

- Fleece lining: It's cozy, breathable, wind-resistant, and fast-drying. But it can be bulky.

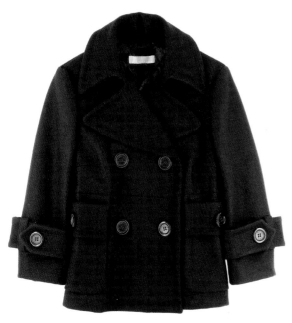

- The hem should be even. Check your side view to be sure.

- A coat needs sway and movement in the back. Use a three-way mirror to make sure yours has both.

- A coat should feel good. Walk around in it for ten minutes. Is the weight comfortable or inhibiting?

- A coat should sit well. Button it up and take a seat in the dressing room. Do the closures pull? Do you have a heavy double flap sitting in your lap?

## THE PERFECT FIT

- Your coat should hang evenly straight down from the shoulders.

- Vents, pleats, pockets, and closures should lie flat.

- Armholes should offer enough room for you to raise your hands over your head without the coat moving up so high that you look like a jack-in-the-box.

- Sleeves should be long enough to cover your wrists.

## LINING

- Look for a substantial lining that's properly finished—no creases or strange tucks. If they've paid attention to the lining, chances are the rest of the coat was made with similar care.

- If you want to make a color statement but shrink from a brightly colored coat, a flash of fuchsia (scarlet, emerald green, acid yellow) lining as you walk will make serious impact.

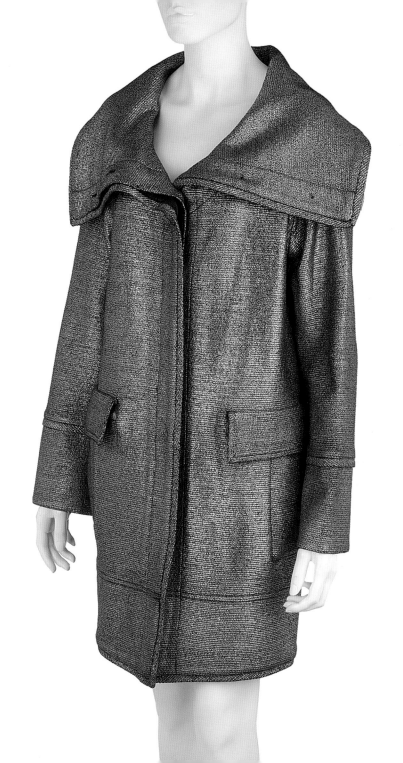

# 8

## HOW TO CHOOSE A
## SUIT

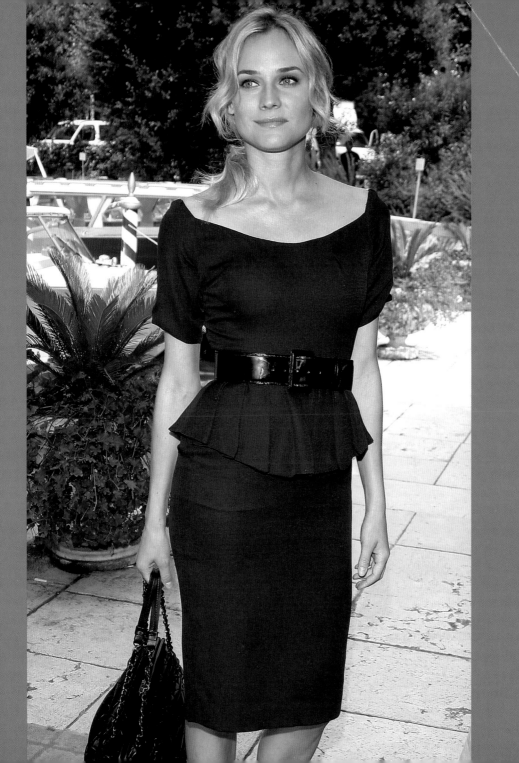

**GIVENCHY SUITS** GAVE ME "PROTECTION"
AGAINST STRANGE SITUATIONS AND PEOPLE,
**BECAUSE I FELT SO GOOD IN THEM.**

Audrey Hepburn

THE SUIT IS FASHION'S equivalent of an Elvis CD. We all own at least one. Whether it reflects your entire lifestyle or just an element of your taste, or is simply something you once thought you ought to have, the suit is the common denominator of modern wardrobes.

If not worn every day, it's still generally our first line of defense when we need to be taken seriously (interviews, business lunches, meetings, presentations). And generally it's also a significant investment.

There's nothing complicated about a suit until you actually get down to choosing one. Whether it's for work, a special occasion, or moral support, it can be one of the most daunting purchases. A lot depends on it making the right impression. A sloppy or badly made suit will impress in all the wrong ways. A well-made suit becomes your backdrop, setting you off as the serenely capable and elegant person you know the world wants to see.

A lot is required of this classic combination. And to complicate matters more, the language of the suit has become so varied. They can be practical, businesslike, dynamic, flirtatious, understated, ironically prim, sleekly refined, or unaccountably seductive.

## SUIT STRATEGY
## FOR EVERY SITUATION

Before you buy, be clear about what you need your suit to do for you. What image are you trying to project? The clearer your goal, the quicker you'll find what you want.

- Who do you want to impress? Your boss, your in-laws, your friends, a judge, yourself?

- What is required of it? Daily duty, moral support, or show-stopping impact?

- Why do you need it? Is it to signal a change of career, a promotion, a new sense of purpose, the steely side of your character?

- Where will you wear it? At the office, on the go, on the town, at a wedding?

- When will you wear it? Often enough to justify a whole new wardrobe of accessories?

## SUIT SENSE

- The best investment starts with the perfect top, and that isn't necessarily a

jacket. Diane Kruger's (on page 151) is a perfect alternative. When you find the top you love, it's worth buying both trousers and a skirt to match it. In one go, you'll maximize your suit's versatility and longevity.

- If you feel your effervescent self is suppressed by the sober suit you have to wear to work, express yourself with a bright lining, but never with novelty items like suspenders or bow ties.

- Avoid boxy jackets under all circumstances. They look heavy and flatter no one. Make sure your waist is defined, if only by the inward curve of the side seams. It doesn't have to be extreme, but even the hint of definition will make a suit look sharper, while a straight drop from armpit to hip has an instant thickening effect.

- Nothing will mire you in middle age faster than chunky fabrics, patch pockets, and buttons masquerading as costume jewelry.

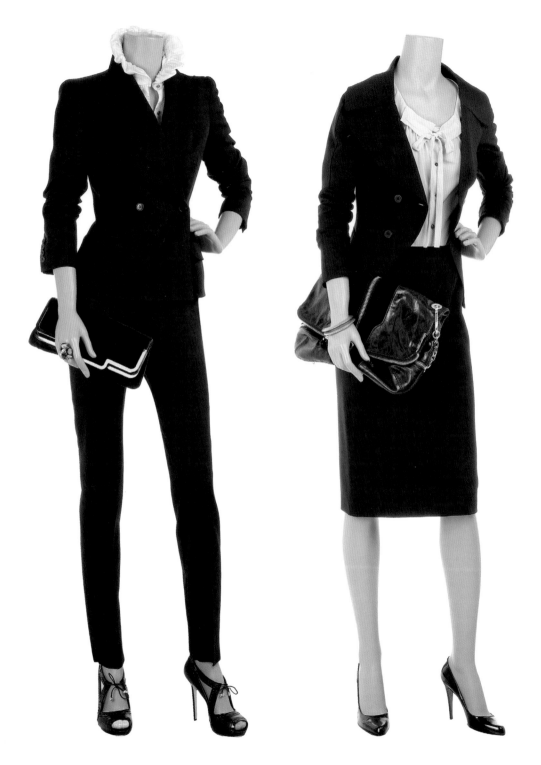

## SUITS ARE SO EASY TO WEAR,

### WHETHER IN A CASUAL OR DRESSY WAY. A WOMAN IN A SUIT IS **THE SEXIEST THING.**

Model Tatjana Patitz in *Harper's Bazaar*

- Nothing ages or dates a suit faster than fussy details. Avoid flouncy peplums, embroidery, wide lapels, intricate pleats, or shoulder pads with a life of their own. If you want to make statements, do it with what you have on underneath and with accessories.

- Flapless pockets look better on everyone.

- Consider a curvy suit with a hint of stretch. The curves deliver impact. The stretch ensures comfort, practical packing, and instant recovery to its sharp and sexy self even after a long-haul flight. At all times think lean, not tight.

- A crisp, lightweight suit is a summer essential. Lined cotton beats linen every time.

- Cost should not be your only indicator of quality. Technology today ensures that a great suit can be found at every price point. What matters more is that it fits and flatters you. To be sure of what a great fit feels like, why not try on an expensive suit and get the benefit of advice from an experienced salesperson? Then apply what you've learned in a shop that better suits your budget.

- Dress to shop in slip-on shoes, unfussy clothes that are easy to get in and out of, silhouette-smoothing underwear, and a neutral-colored shirt, T-shirt, or lightweight sweater. Bring accessories that need to be matched with you, particularly shoes and bags. If the perfect suit you've just found needs new accessories, take it with you when you shop for those.

- Dry cleaning individual pieces separately will ruin your suit.
- Dry-cleaning chemicals are harsh on modern fabrics, so don't send it to the cleaners after every wearing. Try airing instead: A quick spritz with an odor eliminator such as Febreze works wonders. A steamer will be kinder and more efficient than an iron. Isolated stains can be spot treated at home with dry-cleaning pads. Unless you are seriously sloppy with your food or sit next to a cigar smoker, proper dry cleaning twice a season is enough, honestly.

## ALTERATIONS

- You can alter a suit up or down one size at most, but there must be enough fabric in the seams to be able to do that.
- The simplest alterations are length of leg, length of sleeve, and tightness of the waist.
- If a suit needs more than three things altered, put it back and look for something else.

- Trust major alterations only to a qualified tailor.
- If a jacket doesn't fit in the shoulders, take it off at once. Don't believe anyone who says they can fix it.
- Jackets can be taken in at the back center seam, but tailoring side seams is usually less likely to distort the shape and pattern.

## FIGURE NOTES

- Vertical lines created by pinstripes or princess seams will elongate your body.
- If you're worried about your hips, opt for a longer jacket. Wrist-length (or, if you have short arms, hip-length) is the sharpest and most classic length for sizes 8 through 12. Long trousers worn over heels will slim your leg.
- Dark tones create a long line, and a colorful or light-colored top will shift focus to your face.
- Skinny (not tight) sleeves set in a high armhole are fail-safe slimming devices.

- Double-breasted jackets add width, will make a large bust look larger, and overwhelm petite women. What they can do is camouflage a small chest and add power to a boyish figure.

- If you want to go double-breasted, make sure the waist and shoulders are sharply defined. Single-breasted jackets are more flattering on just about everybody. Full busts are most flattered by the deep V-neck of a single-breasted jacket.

- Petites look great in cropped jackets that sit on the waist or the hip bone.

- Eliminating the waistband of a skirt can elongate the body and narrow the line across the hips. If you're short-waisted, try wearing your skirt slightly low-slung (about one inch below the natural waistline). If you're long-waisted, try wearing it one inch above. Just be sure to show a waistline somewhere.

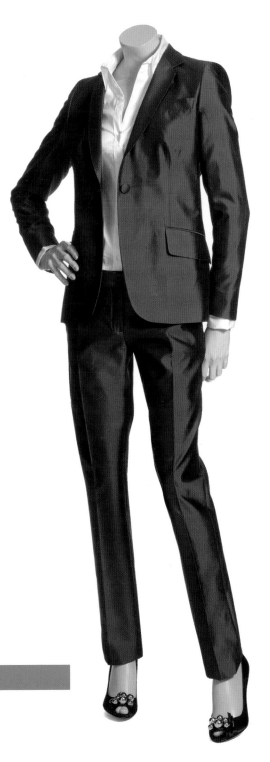

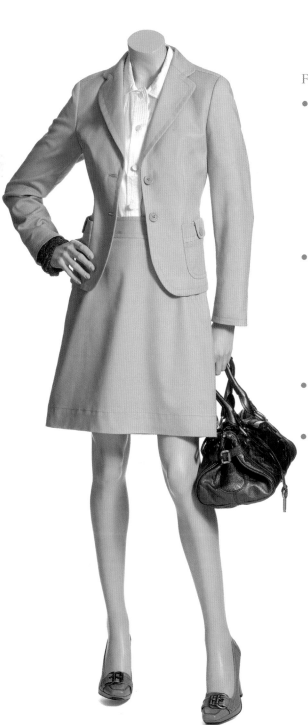

FIT

- A well-cut suit that fits you impeccably is one of the most flattering things you can wear. But think linear and lean, not tight. Expect some restriction of movement. The yoga tree pose might be tough, but hugging yourself shouldn't be.

- A jacket that fits properly should allow you to bend your forearms upward and press your elbows snugly against the front of your body without creating too much strain across the back.

- The back of your collar should be flush with your neck.

- Sleeves that are longer than your wrist have a kind of slouchy attitude, and those that are shortened so they graze the upper part of the wrist bone look great with French-cuffed shirts. These are the limits. Anything shorter will look as if you have grown out of it, and anything below the fleshy part of your thumb will look like your big sister's hand-me-down.

I NEVER LEAVE HOME DRESSED IN ANYTHING **BUT A SUIT.**
**EVEN MORE THAN** A LITTLE BLACK DRESS,
A SUIT GIVES YOU **INSTANT POLISH.**

Model Cordula Reyer in *Harper's Bazaar*

- Suit trousers should be neither too full nor too tight.
- Take advice. A trained salesperson or a tailor will be invaluable to you.

## ANATOMY OF A WELL-MADE JACKET

- LAPEL: A third layer of fabric should be inserted for reinforcement. This is what makes the lapel lie neatly and roll softly.
- BUTTONS: Check how they're sewn on. Having the thread wound around itself between the fabric and the button or around the button's stem makes the connection stronger. Inside the jacket, the button stitching should be hidden inside the lining, leaving nothing visible.
- LINING: The way the lining is made contributes enormously to the fit and comfort of a jacket, so pay careful attention to the finish. It should be made of durable and lightweight fabric such as rayon or silk. It should lie flat and not add any extra weight or bulk. There should be about half an inch of additional lining fabric folded and pressed under at the lining's hem for extra movement. It should not be sewn down anywhere other than the jacket's outer perimeter and armholes. There should be about three inches of the suit's fabric used on the inside flaps running down the front of the jacket.
- SHOULDER: There should be no puckering or unnecessary bulk—even if the shoulder is padded, even if the jacket is inexpensive. Any visible waffling cannot be steamed or pressed out.

# 9

ESSENTIALS: THE PERFECT
PANTS

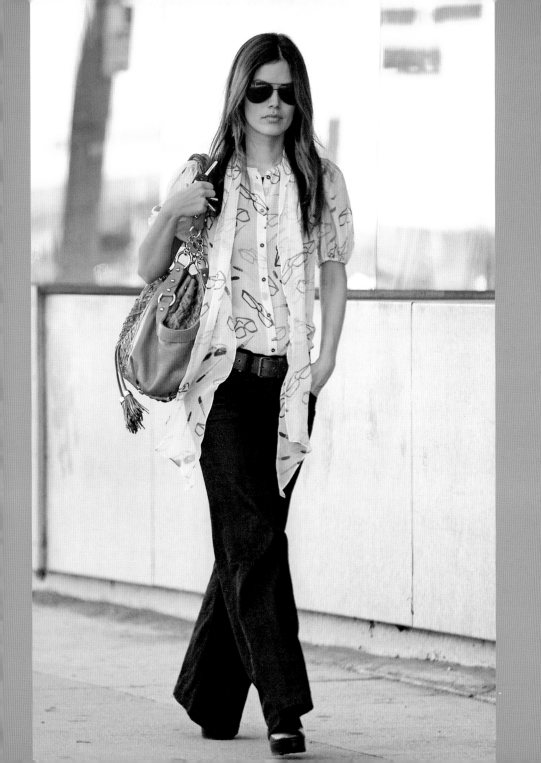

## I WEAR PANTS ALMOST EXCLUSIVELY SO I CAN SIT LIKE A TRUCK DRIVER. I OWN ONE DRESS—A LONG EVENING GOWN.

Lauren Bacall

FOR SO MANY OF US, PANTS ARE a daily staple: We work, party, chill, dance, meet, and travel in them. Get the fit that works and they can be your best friend in your wardrobe—the kind that supports you no matter what you want to be. A great pair of pants can work for you whether you're feeling laid-back or ready to get a job done, glamorous or understated, sexy or girlish, confident and capable, or adolescent and petulant.

It's always been true that one woman's perfect pair of trousers is another's wardrobe crisis. Getting the right fit can take an exhaustive search. There's potential for sag, bag, and ballooning in every tuck and seam. Trousers hug the figure more than dresses or skirts. They highlight the waist, hips, thighs, even calves and ankles. But once you know you have found the right pair for you, whether jeans or tailored trousers, buy in multiples and stick with the brand.

## TEN UNDENIABLE TROUSER TRUTHS (REGARDLESS OF YOUR SHAPE)

1. *Certain proportions will suit your shape better than others.* You need to be sure of what proportion suits you best. A full-length mirror—or better still, a folding three-way one—will be a great help here.

2. *Wide or cropped trousers shorten your leg.* Cuffs shorten even more. Only the very tall

and very slim can wear cuffed pants with flat shoes. Everyone else needs heels.

3. *Getting the length right is at least as important as whether your butt looks big or not.* So when you try trousers on or have alterations done, do it with the type of shoe you intend to wear. For a classic length, the back of your trouser leg should clear the floor by a quarter inch, and the instep should be covered with the front grazing the top of your shoe. If you'll be wearing the trousers with different heel heights, leave an extra one-eighth-inch of fabric in the length to accommodate the higher shoes. But remember, there is a limit to the versatility of one length. Don't expect it to work perfectly with both your highest heels *and* your flats. For those extremes, you need different pairs of pants.

4. *In general, avoid pockets with flaps.* The extra detail just adds width. Flapless pockets are more streamlined and look better on anyone.

5. *Steer clear of pleated trousers unless you have one of those tummies that caves in.* Flat-front trousers look better every time.

6. *Floral-printed trousers are not a good look in the city.* If you must have a pair, wear them (with a solid-colored top) on holiday. If you want to wear printed trousers in the city, go for something more geometric, such as a '50s or '60s print. Bridget Riley's modernist prints, Marimekko's wood-blocked flowers, Pucci's psychedelic swirls, or Damien Hirst's dots also look great in the summer in the city. Once again, keep the top simple.

7. *Animal-print pants are over.* Even Rod Stewart has put away his leopard print leggings. Need I say more? Restrict your zoological urges to other parts of your body.

8. *White trousers in winter look great.* Just stick to a heavy fabric, something like wool, flannel, cashmere, or a tweedy weave. Opt for a shade tinged with ivory to soften the starkness of the white, which might look a touch cold in winter light. Wear them with a cream, black, camel, or gray turtleneck and a dark suede or animal-print shoe. In winter, white trousers and white shoes are fine if you

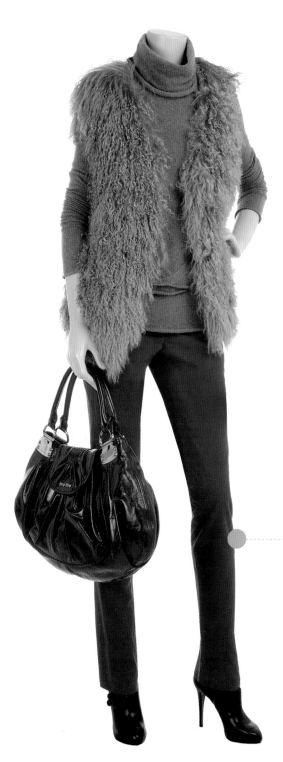

are going for a retro look. If all you want is a pale shoe, a reptile skin is a more versatile neutral in this case.

9. *If cropped trousers shorten your leg too much, don't wear them just because everyone else is.* Similarly, avoid low-slung pants if they emphasize your tummy's bulge.

10. *Heels worn under pants will give a brilliant boost your to you rear view.*

## TRICKY TROUSER SHAPES

More and more, different trouser shapes—that all require particular shoes, accessories, and tops—are becoming classics. Here's a quick rundown of what works with what . . . and what doesn't.

### LOW-RISE BOOT CUT

- Always wear low-waisted trousers with a top that is long enough to cover both your tummy and behind. Or have a slim top that skims the upper half of the body to the waist and sits neatly inside

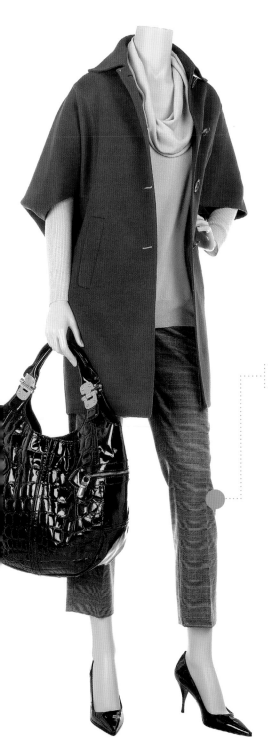

your waistband (slim polo-neck sweater, vest top, slim-cut shirt or T-shirt). High heels will add the extra inches the low-slung waist has taken away, and make sure your trousers are long enough to "break" on the top of your shoes.

- Figure warning: No matter how perfect your figure, anything that blouses out over the top of your waistband will look like you are trying to hide a paunch or maybe a pregnancy.

## CROPPED

- If the trousers hit below the knee, try them with high boots in the same color for the longest leg possible. Make sure there is no gap between the top of the boot and bottom of the trousers, even when you are sitting down. Or try high-heeled shoes and opaque tights. A slightly chunky cut with a round toe and stacked heel works better than pointy.

- If you minimize the top half of your body with a narrow jacket or a slim-fitting

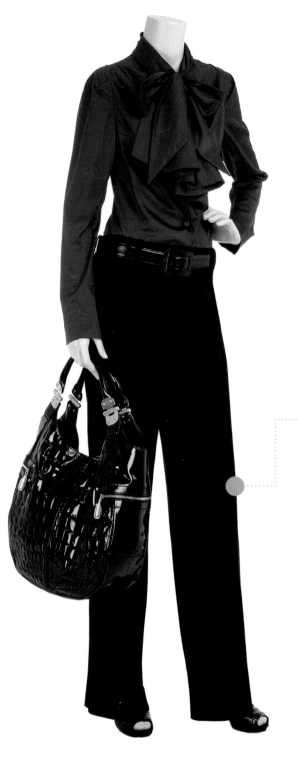

sweater, you'll get extra height, too. A slouchy sweater makes this a great weekend look.

- Evening-weight or decorative fabrics will look great with high-heeled evening shoes with an ankle strap.

- Figure warning: If you're short and slim, keep your cropped trousers slim-legged, your top slim-fitting, and your heels high to avoid being shortened further. If you are small and curvy, don't try this look, even at home.

## HIGH OR LOW WAIST WITH WIDE LEGS

Trousers that sit above your natural waistline are good leg lengtheners, so if you love to wear flats, go get 'em.

- For the long-legged, straight, wide-legged trousers with a cummerbund or Japanese obi-style belt making a high waist will look great with flat shoes and make a particularly good evening option (useful if you are a hostess with lots of running

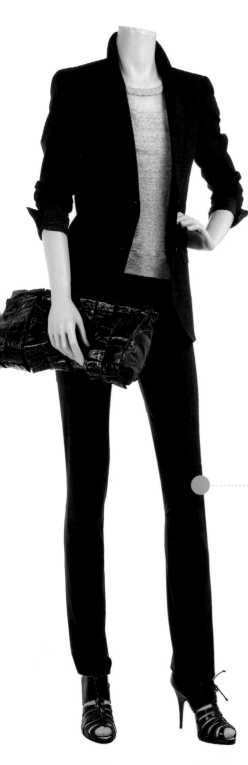

around to do). Choose a pair the same color as your trousers.

- For smaller women who love a wide-legged look, a low-waisted pant worn with a slight heel will keep your legs from looking stumpy. With any wide-legged pants, either keep the top slim-fitting or limit any volume to fine-gauge knit or drapey fabric. Stilettoes look too delicate under voluminous cuffs. On the other hand, a platform stacked-heel sandal would look fabulous.

- Figure warning: If you have short legs or a bottom that is large in proportion to your waist, the low-waist look is not for you.

## SKINNY LEG

The key here is balance.

- A chunky sweater that covers your hips and high heels will make your legs look longer and leaner and is terrific if you have great legs and a curvy upper half.

- A narrow, fitted jacket and stilettos are all rock 'n' roll attitude but suitable only for the leanest limbed.

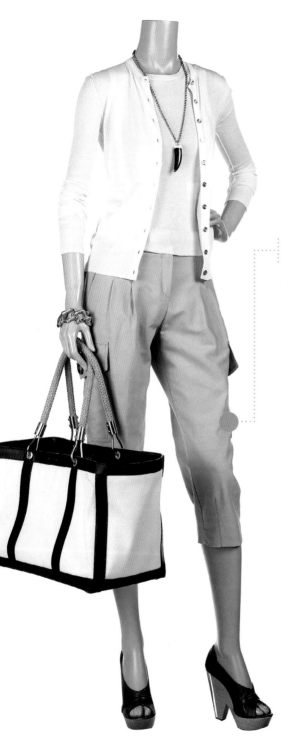

- For some uptown gloss, go for a top with some volume or structure and a high, skinny heel.
- Figure warning: Don't wear flat shoes with skinny pants unless you are a size 4 or under.

## CARGO PANTS

Just when you thought it was safe to get into your classic black trousers again, those darn cargo pants make a comeback, fully loaded with zips, flaps, pockets, and more potential style mistakes than you'll find outside a political convention. This is not fashion for the fainthearted, but there are ways to get that hipness to work for you.

- Keep the top slim: could be a narrow tailored jacket, a slim-cut shirt, or even a T-shirt and sleeveless jacket. Avoid a bare midriff unless you are totally toned. Cargo pants need a high heel. It can be chunky, skinny, strappy . . . whatever.
- Remember: You need to make a judgment call about every new look based on what works for you and your

body. Just because everybody is doing something doesn't mean it looks good. They may just be storing up fashion memories that, in ten years' time, will make little children laugh.

- Figure warning: Cargo pants look great with flat shoes only on twentysomethings whose bouncy youth protects them from the volume added by thigh flaps and flip-flops. Anyone older needs to balance that width with height.

## STRAIGHT-LEGGED, FLAT-FRONT

- This is a classic mariner cut, and it's a great weekend alternative to jeans or cargo pants. It will look great with chunky heels but is also very cute with sneakers.
- Try a figure-skimming sweater or a straight-cut tunic that sits on the hip (a stripey sailor shirt will never be a cliché ).
- Figure warning: A high waist in this shape will do nothing for your butt or your legs. Think Simon Cowell—need I say more? A waist that sits on your hip bone is as high as you should go.

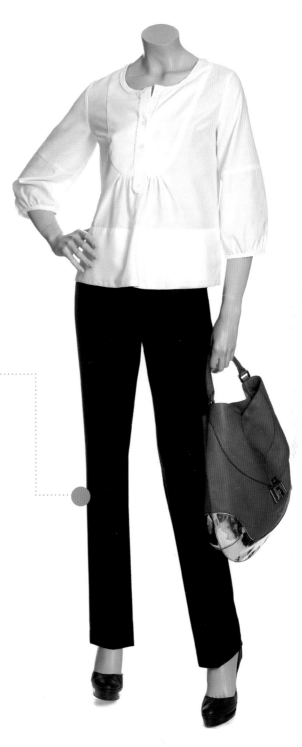

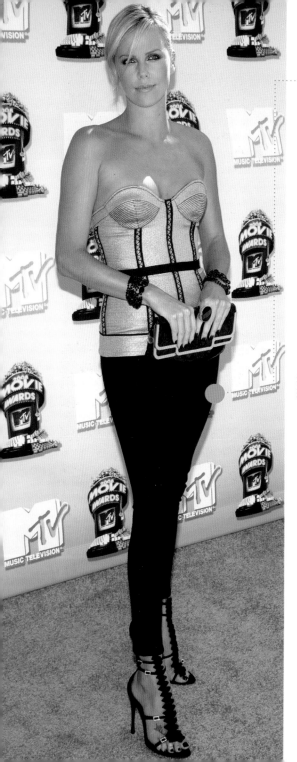

## LEGGINGS

- Under a dress or hip-covering tunic, fine—as long as they hit below the bulge of your calf. On their own? Only if you are twelve or have the legs of a twelve-year-old. For anyone else, they are only right for the gym.

- Figure warning: Fat, slim, tall, short—these can look pretty terrible on just about anyone with knees. You're in treacherous fashion territory. Watch out!

## PLEAT-FRONT TROUSERS

Aaaaaaaaagh! Of all the trousers ever made, these are the toughest to carry off, and yet they never go or stay away for long. Approach them with extreme caution.

- Curvy women in particular should react like a vampire to garlic.

- Contrary to popular opinion, they do not camouflage unwanted curves—they accentuate them.

- Be my guest, if you're a 5'7" beanpole. Everyone else: flat-front trousers only, please.

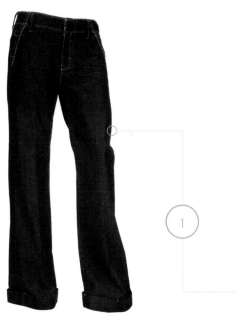

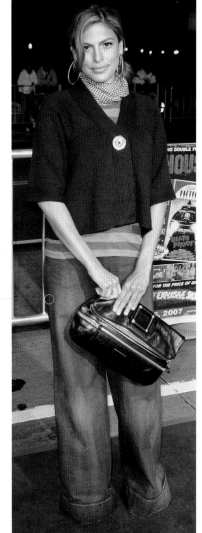

① ①

## JEANS—GET THE PERFECT FIT FOR YOUR FIGURE!

### 1. Voluptuous Curves

- Classic or relaxed fits are best. They'll give you ease and flattery in the bottom area without being big all over.

- Get a pair that sits on your hips rather than your waist.

- Concentrate on getting the waist and leg proportion just right. Get it wrong and you just make your bottom look bigger. The waistband should sit just below your waist's natural curve and the leg should skim your natural shape. A waist-cinching shape with lots of fabric in the leg is about the worst thing you can do for your figure.

- Figure warning: Avoid too-tight legs and small or widely spaced back pockets. These things all add width.

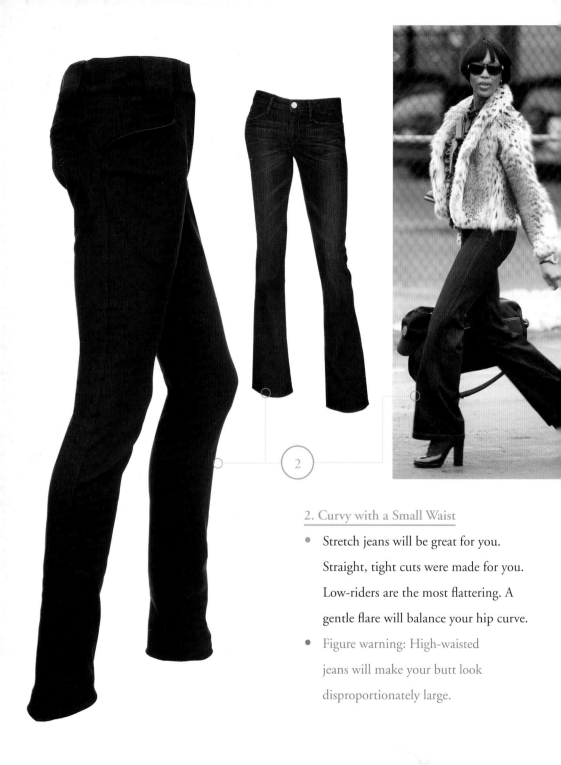

## 2. Curvy with a Small Waist

- Stretch jeans will be great for you. Straight, tight cuts were made for you. Low-riders are the most flattering. A gentle flare will balance your hip curve.
- Figure warning: High-waisted jeans will make your butt look disproportionately large.

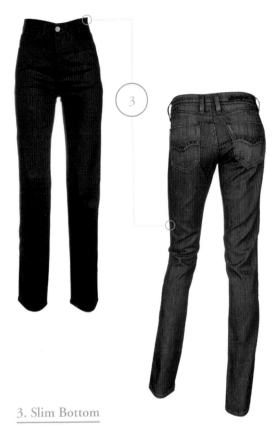

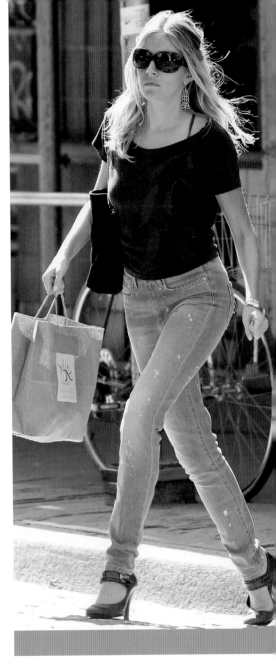

## 3. Slim Bottom

- Stretch jeans, but not second-skin tight, are best. Go for a slim leg. They hug, defining any curves you have. Back pockets, for you alone, can be as decorative as you want. Flaps? Even better.

- Figure warning: Avoid stiff denim, boy cuts, and baggy, loose fits.

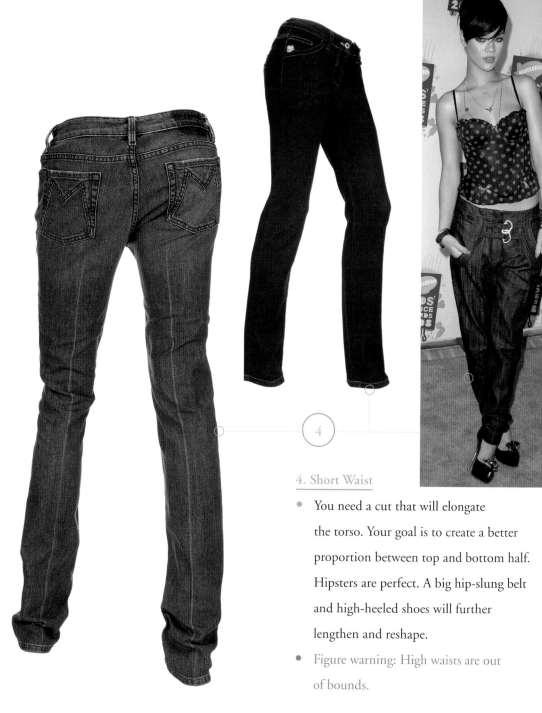

### 4. Short Waist

- You need a cut that will elongate
  the torso. Your goal is to create a better
  proportion between top and bottom half.
  Hipsters are perfect. A big hip-slung belt
  and high-heeled shoes will further
  lengthen and reshape.

- Figure warning: High waists are out
  of bounds.

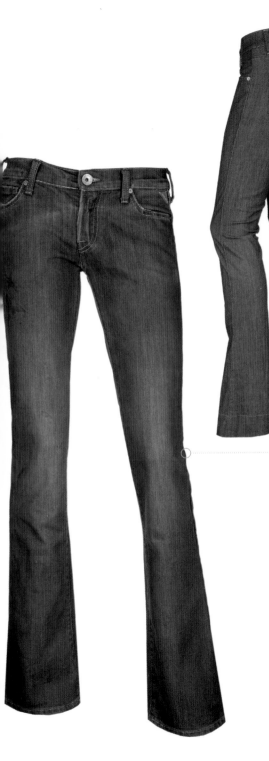

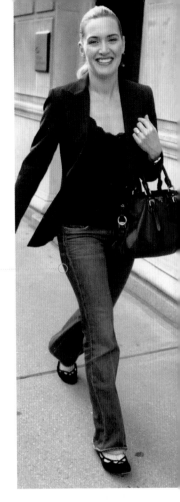

### 5. Heavy Thighs

- An easy fit on the hips is key. Avoid tapered legs and anything oversize.
- Boot-legs help balance the heaviness further up.
- Don't tuck tops in, but keep the silhouette neat to avoid the baggy look.
- Figure warning: High, tight waists will exaggerate thigh width. Avoid at all costs.

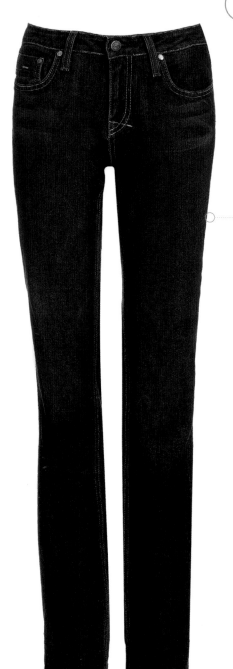

 6

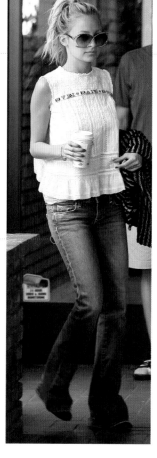

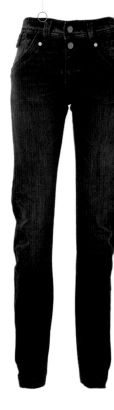

### 6. Petite with Short Legs

- You need to lengthen your legs and add curve to your figure. A waist that sits on or just above the hip, cut with straight legs, adds length. Wear heels and make sure your hem is long enough to break but not fold over on the top of your foot.

- Figure warning: Low-cut jeans and wide legs will both rob you of precious inches.

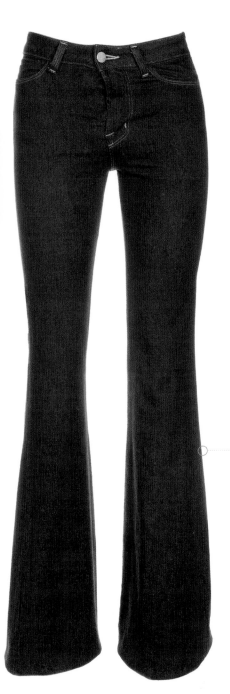

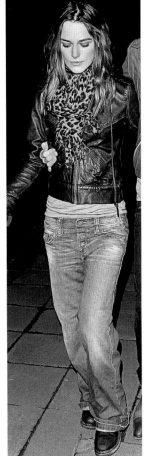

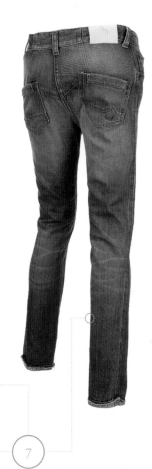

7

### 7. Long Waist

- You need to shorten your torso and lengthen your legs.
- Wear jeans that hit your natural waist and have snug-fitting legs. The narrow cut will lengthen further. Add more height by going for a long leg and wearing heels.
- Figure warning: Avoid ankle-cropped lengths.

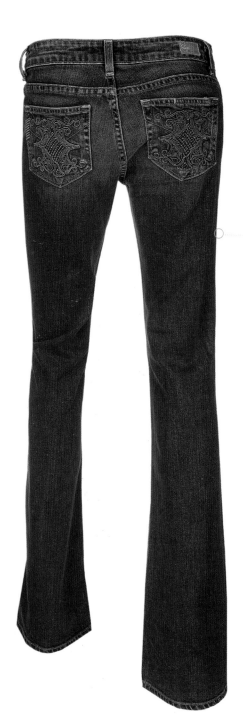

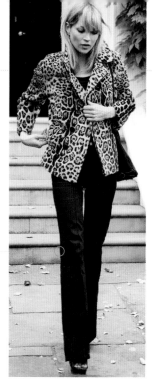

### 8. Boyish Figure

- For the slim-hipped and straight-waisted, it's essential to add curve and definition to your figure. Experiment between a high-waisted pair and a low-rise, straight-leg jean. The boy cut is great for you. Add big sweaters and flat shoes for a gamine beatnik look. Or try a sexy shirt and high heels to be more sophisticated.

- Figure warning: Success is all in getting the waist that optimizes your curves. Get that right and pretty much any leg will look great on you.

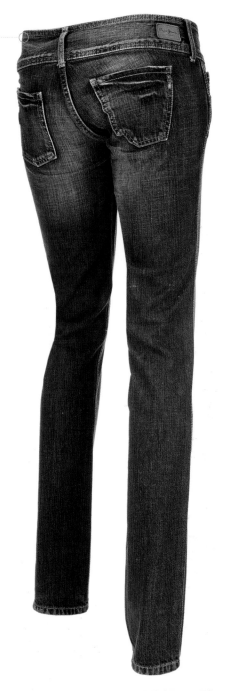

BY THE WAY:
A WORD ON YOUR REAR

Jeans look best in a medium- to heavyweight denim. Thinner fabric will highlight, not hide, bulges. Judge denim's weight by handling. It should feel substantial.

# 10

## ESSENTIALS: THE IDEAL
## D R E S S

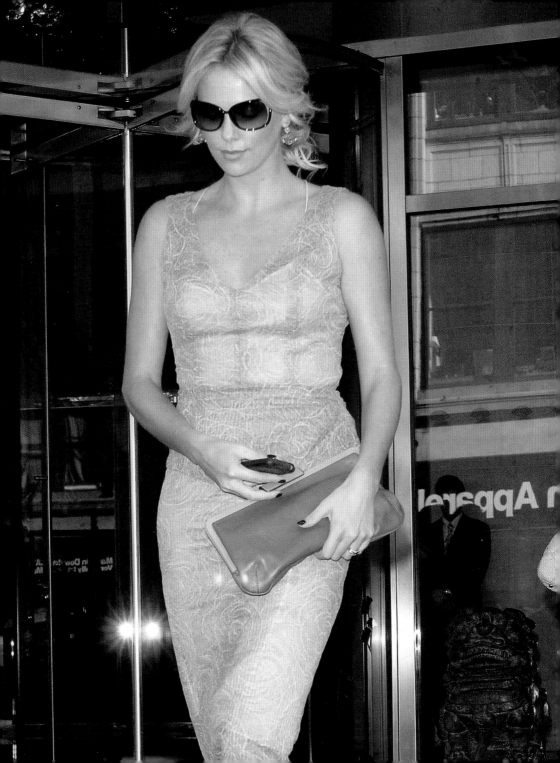

# A WOMAN DOES NOT SIMPLY WEAR A DRESS: SHE LIVES IN IT.

Hubert de Givenchy

EVER WISHED YOU COULD find the emergency exit in a wardrobe crisis? Generations of stylish women, looking for the most direct route out of a fashion dilemma, have known that you can depend on a dress. It's a one-hit wonder—all you need are shoes and you're ready to go. Sure, you can accessorize as much as you like, but even with the most minimal styling, a great dress can make you look polished and pulled together in an instant.

In the twenty-first century, the dress gets two reactions: One is devotion, and the other is "over my dead body." For many, it's still a throwback to those ladylike days before denim, when bags matched shoes and no one stepped out without gloves. For others, it's always been too difficult to find the dress that best suits their body shape.

Separates now form the backbone of most modern wardrobes. And, compared to our grandmothers, most women have a much more freewheeling approach to getting their look together. But if you're trying to edit some of the chaos out of your life, it may just be worth taking another look at the practical benefits of one-piece dressing.

A tailored shift will segue easily from work to the cocktail hour. A simple column in cotton or silk looks crisper and fresher in summer than layers of separates. And the fluidity of jersey or crepe delivers elegance with an edge.

The right dress can add height, broaden your shoulders, and skim your hips. You can vamp it up, play it down, or simply enjoy the pure feminine pleasure in a swish of fabric or a nipped-in waist.

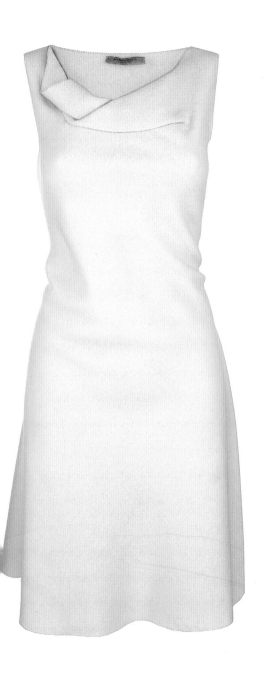

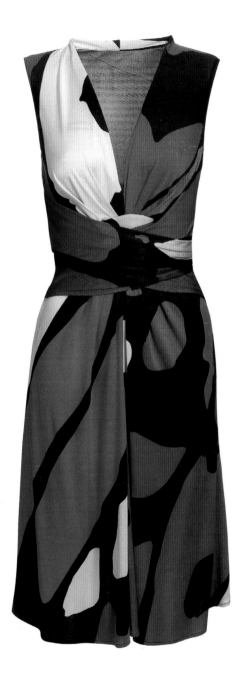

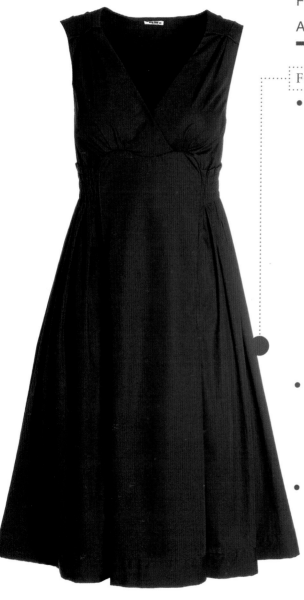

## THE RIGHT DRESS:
## FOR WORK, FOR THE WEEKEND,
## AND FOR EVENING

### FOR WORK

- Keep it simple. A tailored shape is best in most office situations. That doesn't mean it has to be a shift, if that does not work for your figure. It could just as easily be a shirtdress (adds curves where there aren't any, disguises the tummy, sharpens shoulders, defines the waist, and, if V-necked, also lengthens the torso). A tailored A-line is another great option (particularly good for disguising wide-hipped figures).

- If you need to cover up, say for formal meetings and presentations, go for a jacket that echoes the line of the dress. A boxy jacket kills a curvy dress.

- Consider a cardigan for a softer, more feminine option. Keep it sleek (fine-knit lamb's wool, cotton, silk, or cashmere). Keep the buttons discreet (small pearl buttons are always great). All bets are off if the cardigan once belonged to your dad or boyfriend.

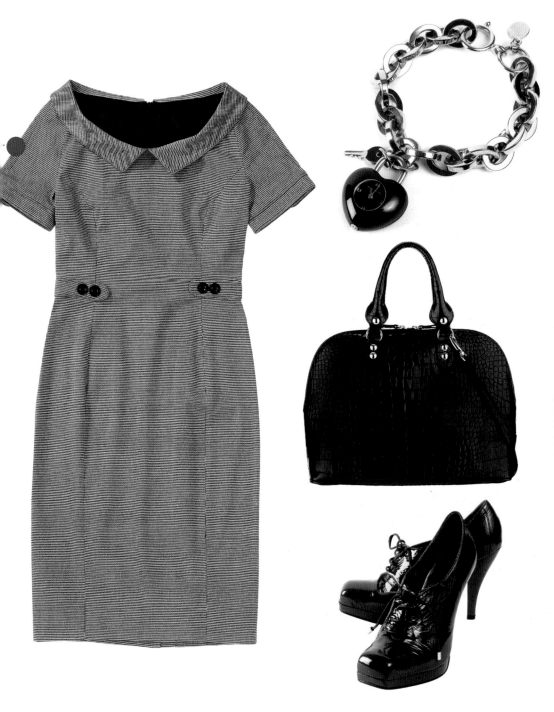

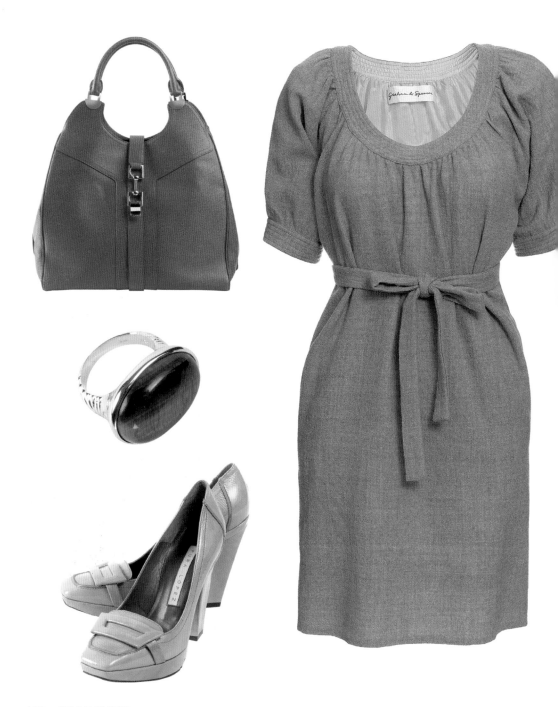

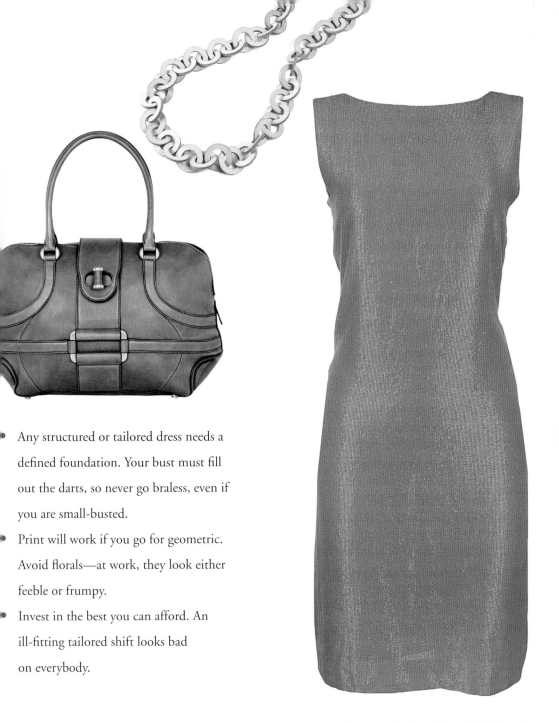

- Any structured or tailored dress needs a defined foundation. Your bust must fill out the darts, so never go braless, even if you are small-busted.

- Print will work if you go for geometric. Avoid florals—at work, they look either feeble or frumpy.

- Invest in the best you can afford. An ill-fitting tailored shift looks bad on everybody.

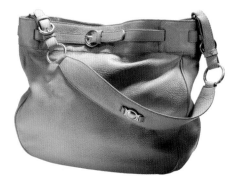

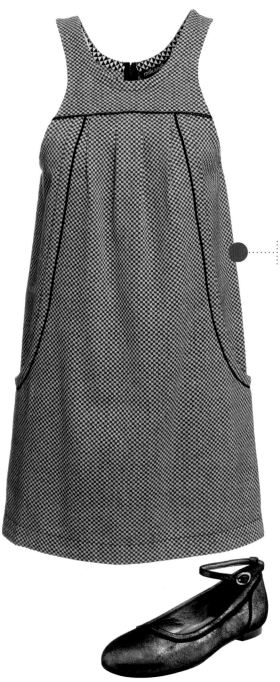

- Keep shapes simple: Your only priority for your time out should be to minimize fuss.

- Cotton (poplin, pique, lawn, shirting), denim, or jersey should be your fabrics of choice.

- Make free with print and bright color. If exuberant print and color make you happy, you can get away with them now.

- Buy cheaply. Quantity wins out over quality here: between beach days, country weekends, lunch with the girls, and city shopping trips, it's good to have options and to be able to wear, trash, and move on.

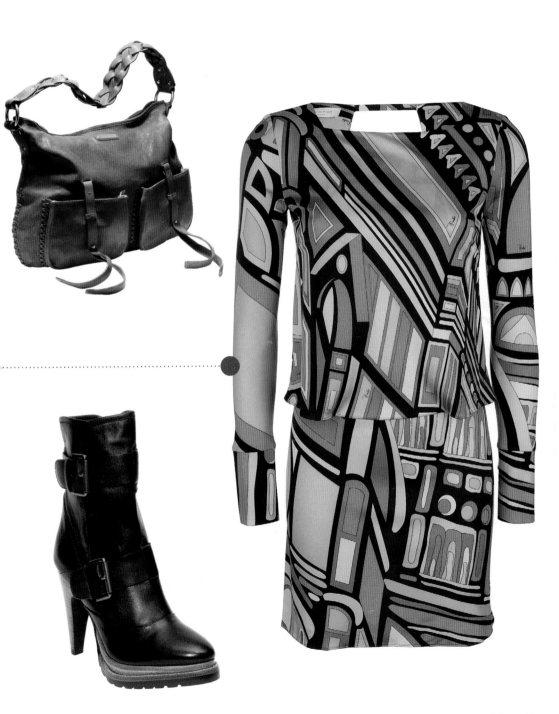

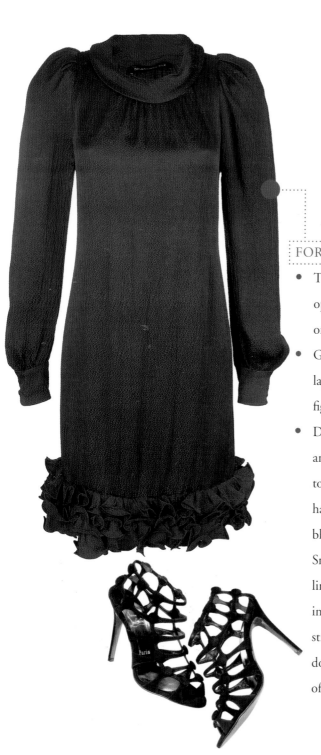

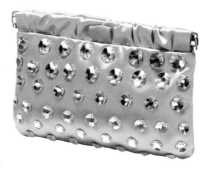

FOR EVENING

- The little black dress is everyone's favorite option (see below), but it isn't the only one.

- Go for lingerie details: lace trims, chiffon layers, even bias-cut charmeuse (if your figure can take its merciless exposure).

- Dark colors are just as versatile as black and often more flattering, particularly to very pale or freckly skins with light hair color. Check out plum, midnight blues, garnet reds, and chocolate browns. Smoky grays, metallics, and pinks are lingerie staples that also deliver glamour in the evening because they make a strong statement. Remember, the downside of this is that the wardrobe life of the big statement can be limited.

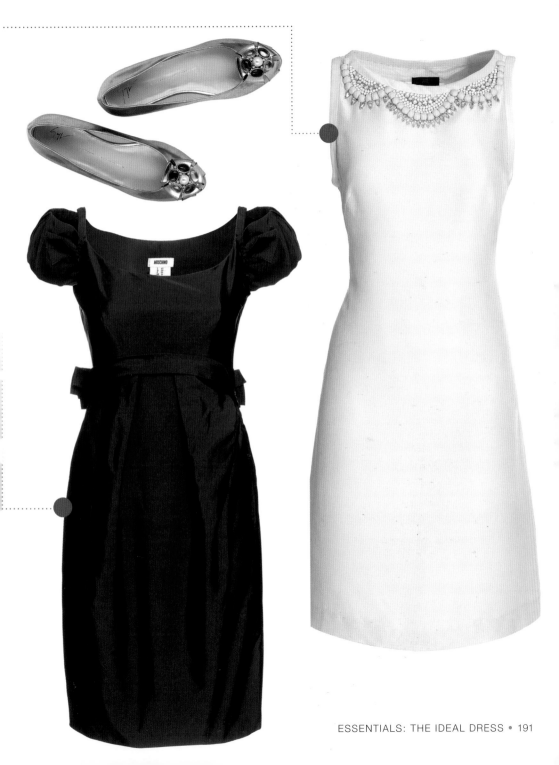

## CHOOSING THE BEST DRESS FOR YOUR FIGURE

- Pear-shaped figures will really benefit from the defining and smoothing effects of a sharp-shouldered, bias-cut style.
- A-lines are the best hip minimizers.
- The best necklines for large bosoms are the boatneck, V-neck, keyhole, or square. Avoid round necks, high necks, or turtlenecks. Reverse and shawl collars are also slimming and lengthening. Stick to fitted, body-skimming silhouettes, and avoid crossover styles that cut your bosom in two at all costs.
- A curvy figure looks best in fabrics that drape rather than cling. Never leave your waist undefined. Even the subtlest curve in at the waist will look better than a boxy drop from the shoulder that will only add width.
- An hourglass shape with a full skirt and nipped-in waist will give boyish figures some feminine oomph.

- A tailored, waisted shift will subtly shape a boyish frame.
- A curvy figure will stop traffic in a wrap dress.
- Heavy arms can be disguised by slim (not tight) three-quarter length sleeves.
- Empire waists lengthen petite frames.
- An all-over print keeps the eye moving and disguises a multitude of figure faults.

## HOW TO GET THE BEST FIT

- Dresses can be tricky because they have to fit well in so many different spots: shoulders, waist, hips, bust, and length. Here's where label loyalty pays off. Try lots of different designers, and when you find one whose cut works for you, stick with it.
- Add definition with a belt. Even if your dress is seamed at the waist, that may not be enough. The addition of something as simple as a grosgrain ribbon in a contrasting or toning color, tied in a bow at your waist, could be the only thing that separates the dynamic from the droopy.

- In the fitting room, make sure you can sit down, cross your legs, bend over and reach up without pinching or squeezing (which will make you look bigger than you are) or exposing more than you want to.

- A tailor can reasonably be expected to adjust hem length (up or down), shoulder width (narrower is easier than wider), strap length, or waist width (in is easier than out). If more than one of these is required, you're probably buying the wrong size or style of dress. No tailor can make a dress grow to accommodate a butt or bust that is too big for it.

## THE LITTLE BLACK DRESS

There's probably no single item of clothing that is more useful (okay, okay, jeans queens, you have a point). When you need to make an impression, nothing disguises pounds or adds height and general allure like the little black dress. Its detractors argue that its inherent chicness is often canceled out by its dull blackness. Frankly, those who think that

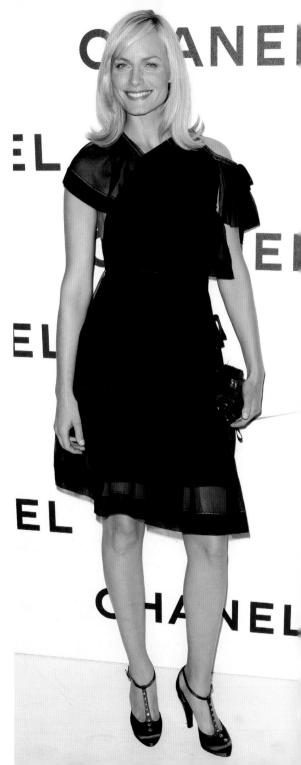

a perfectly tailored and minimally adorned dress is a head turner at any event are still in the majority. However, if you feel you need to alleviate the density, pay attention to the detail: stitched pleats, asymmetrical necklines, seaming, soft frills and lace, or chiffon overlays are all effective.

If you're making the best of a cut-price dress, then the simpler the better. In this case, avoid fussy details like bows, frills, and beading at all costs, and remember: scratchy, synthetic lace is style poison.

The best length hits your knee just below the crinkly part. If you have fabulous knees (and there really are not many of them about, so be brutally honest with yourself), your hem can settle a few inches higher without losing any of that LBD sleek chic. Another gorgeous length, particularly if you've gone for an A-line skirt, is three-quarter length. Just be sure the hem hits below the calf's widest part or it will thicken and shorten your leg.

Clearly, the little black dress is not as simple as it looks. Any old one will not do.

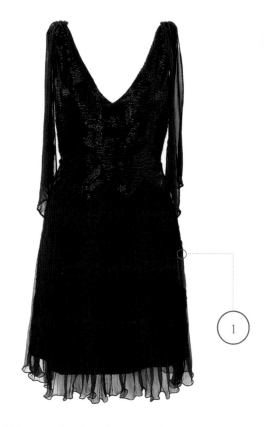

When you're choosing, consider how to make your own unique impact. What are your figure's focal points?

1. Great neck and shoulders? A wide V-backed dress could be a stunning alternative to those strapless or off-the-shoulder staples. Focusing the attention at the nape of your neck will have major impact. Put long hair up to maximize your style advantage.

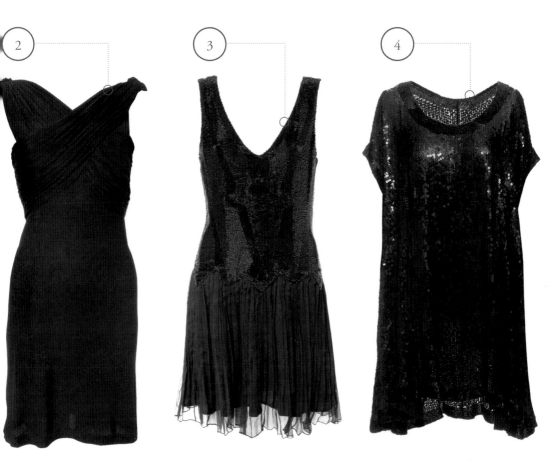

2. Boyish figure? You're one of the few who can get away with a simple shift. Create curves with a belt or seaming at the waist. A sleeveless dress that's slightly cut away at the shoulder line will also strengthen your look. You can also get away with ruffles and frills, which are figure-killers on just about any other body type.

3. Large bust? A V-neck will balance your curves. Make sure there's good support built in. You also need to keep the overall silhouette under control and avoid billowing fabrics.

4. Great legs? A mini length is not necessarily the most versatile LBD. A hem that hits your knee with a flippy little detail or a floaty fabric that plays when you move (such as chiffon) is way more seductive.

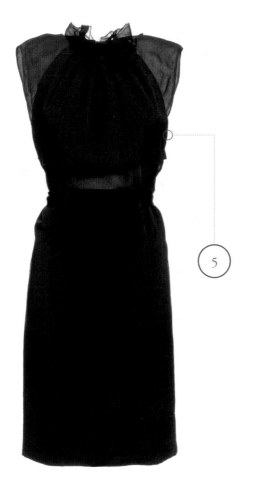

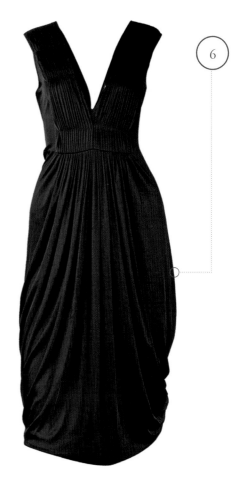

5. No bust? A pleated, frilled, beaded, or corseted bodice will define your top half.

6. Voluptuous curves with a waist? A corseted dress is likely to look delicious on you. Don't be afraid to bare a shoulder. A wide V-neck that skims your collarbones is enough. And, if you want to disguise hips, too, keep the fabric fluid and the skirt silhouette soft.

7. Voluptuous curves and no waist? A tailored A-line is the most flattering shape. Go for a length just below the

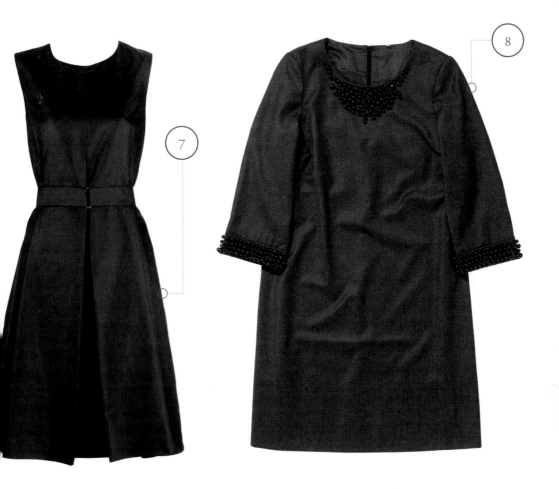

knee to get as much height as possible.
And, once again, drawing the eye up
to an exposed shoulder is a great
balancing trick. If you don't want to bare
a shoulder, a great piece of jewelry at the
neckline (either a brooch or necklace)
will be as effective.

8. Full hips? A figure-skimming A-line
with a plunging neckline (doesn't have to
be too deep) will draw the eye up
and give you good camouflage. Choose
a fabric that moves. Anything too stiff
will undermine your best effort.

- It has to have a heel. Even a low kitten heel is better than none at all. Yes, Audrey Hepburn did look divine in a ballerina-length black dress and ballet flats, but she had the body of a fourteen-year-old at the time. If you have a regular, grown woman's body, just don't go there.

- Black silk slingbacks should be part of every woman's wardrobe. They are the most versatile evening shoe by far. Leather will work, at a push, but to kill the daytime feeling, it should have some strappy detail.

- Strappy evening shoes look great with the LBD. Their delicacy is a perfect foil for all the blackness. If you go open-toed and strappy, be prepared to go bare-legged, and get a pedicure. Never wear pantyhose.

- If you need to wear tights, go for a close-toed shoe and opt for the light coverage of a sheer stocking or fishnet. The blackness from shoulder to knee needs balancing with a light leg to keep it from looking funereal.

- The simpler the dress, the more elaborate the shoes can be. Go for it with red satin, metallic leather, jeweled straps, embroidered velvet. Almost any color will look good as long as it is strong; insipid pastels don't stand up to black.

- Evening boots can look great, but your black dress should be in a winter weight fabric: cashmere, heavy jersey, or velvet.

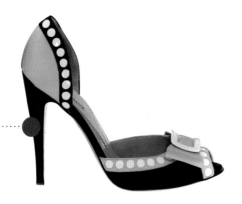

## JEWELRY

Your LBD can take the exuberance of baroque chandelier earrings. But it will also gain strength from the simplest stud. The choice is yours.

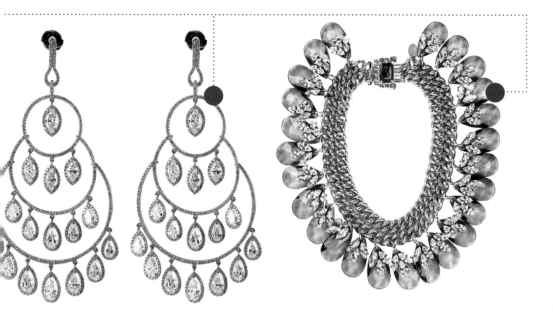

However, if you go for a dramatic jewelry statement, limit it to one. The gorgeous pin will only fight with the dramatic cuffs and the heirloom necklace and, behind them all, your LBD will look like an afterthought. The success of this dress lies in its simplicity. Never overaccessorize.

## WRAPS

If you need to cover up, a shawl is probably the most practical option. However, it is borderline boring. Consider the options of:

- A sharply tailored jacket: a great 1940s

combination that delivers vampy glamour. Keep it feminine. Curvy tailored shapes work better with your LBD than masculine angles.

- An evening coat: a great evening wardrobe investment. Go for embroidered velvets, beaded wools, or dramatic satins. They'll all look gorgeous with your little black dress and just about anything else you want to glam up for the evening, from jeans to a floor-length gown. A fine-gauge cashmere cardigan is a simple but effectively chic cover up.

# 11

## ESSENTIALS: THE SKIRT FOR ALL SEASONS

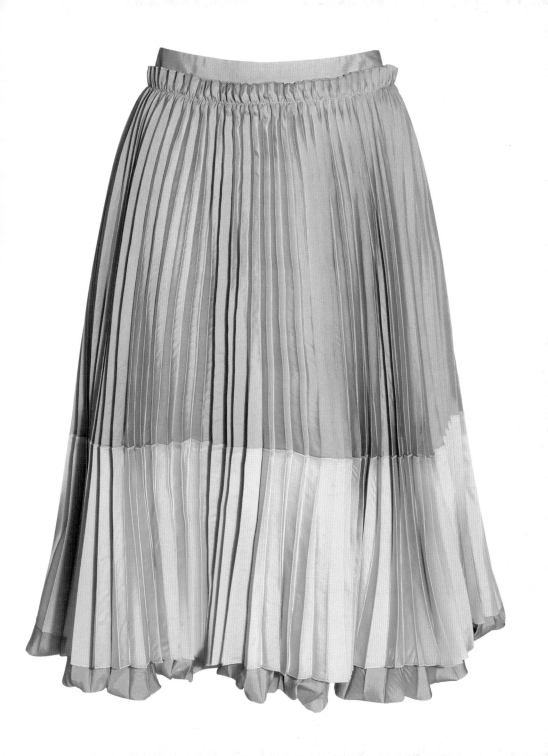

## IF YOU ARE **AT A LOSS WHAT TO WEAR,** **TRY A FITTED JACKET** AND A STRAIGHT SKIRT. **IT'S NEARLY FOOLPROOF.**

Betty Halbreich, director of personal shopping services at Bergdorf Goodman and author of *Secrets of a Fashion Therapist*

THERE ARE WOMEN WHO LOVE to wear skirts and there are those who swear by the practicality of pants. And, as fashion tribes go, they are as separate as church and state. Love it or hate it, the skirt is still regulation uniform in offices that insist on a formal dress code. And, in the evening, the right skirt signals the party spirit better than almost any other single garment.

The skirt gets bad press when fashion goes sporty. True, a skirt doesn't have the same kicked-back ease as a pair of jeans, and it doesn't begin to measure up to the tomboy freedom of your khakis. But, trouser gals, consider this: Can you imagine a departing view of Marilyn Monroe ever delivering the same jaw-dropping impact in a pair of cargo pants? As soon as a little sexy glamour is called for, a great skirt should be your first port of call.

If every skirt you've ever tried on made you feel like a sausage poured into a too-tight skin, maybe you just haven't found the right one yet.

# THE RIGHT SKIRT:
# FOR WORK, FOR THE WEEKEND,
# AND FOR EVENING

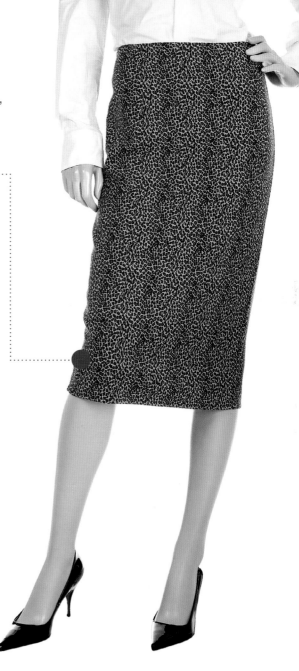

## FOR WORK

- The two key shapes are a simple, tailored A-line or a body-skimming pencil skirt. They are strong separates on their own, looking sharp with just a simple shirt, T-shirt, or fine-knit sweater. But add a jacket and, when the need arises, they get serious in a second.

- Leather skirts can look good in the office as long as they say sleek chic, not biker babe. Heavy metal details, distressed finishes, or a skirt that sags at the seat when you are standing up just doesn't cut it at work.

- The most versatile winter fabrics are tropical wools and wool crepes.

- In the summer, opt for a good-quality cotton that can hold its shape and not go limp and wrinkly the moment the mercury rises.

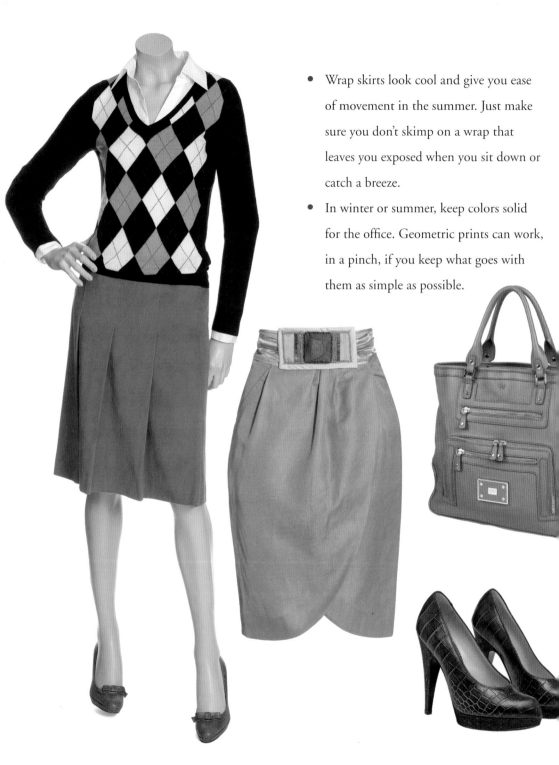

- Wrap skirts look cool and give you ease of movement in the summer. Just make sure you don't skimp on a wrap that leaves you exposed when you sit down or catch a breeze.
- In winter or summer, keep colors solid for the office. Geometric prints can work, in a pinch, if you keep what goes with them as simple as possible.

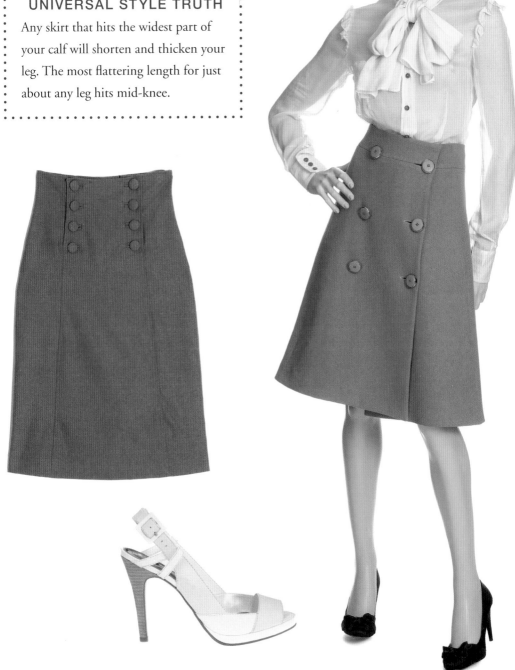

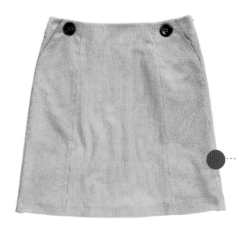

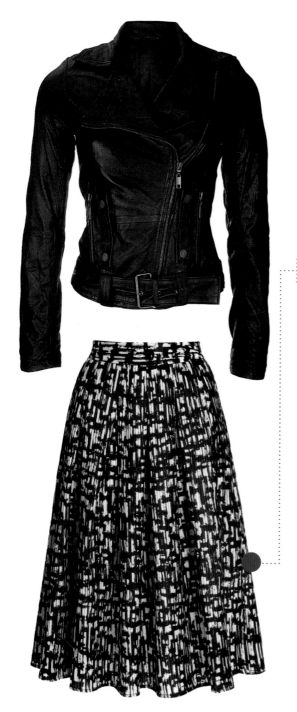

## FOR THE WEEKEND

- Denim, corduroy, or chino skirts are a great alternative to jeans and khakis for the weekend, year-round. Reserve the floaty florals for the summertime.

- Suede is one of the most high-maintenance materials around. No matter what they tell you, the product has not yet been invented to prevent it from permanently absorbing every splash and smudge. This makes them too stressful for anyone who is often in the company of small children or sloppy waiters. If you can avoid all of the above, a suede skirt can add some luxury to your weekend look.

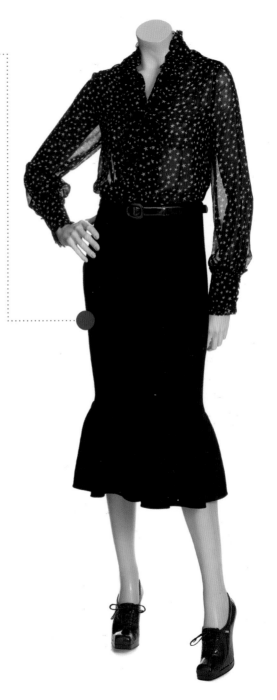

## LONG SKIRTS FOR DAY

- This is a great way to hide a heavy leg. If you're tall, you can wear it skimming the floor with flat shoes or ankle-length with boots.

- Petites are better off with three-quarter length skirts over tall high-heeled boots.

- The long skirt can look sleek without sacrificing height if you keep the volume under control.

- A long skirt is also an unexpectedly breezy and cool option for summer.

## MINISKIRTS

- If you have ample hips, avoid miniskirts at all costs. They focus attention right where you don't want it.

- If you're nowhere near a beach, there are generally only a few inches of skin between the sleek and the cheap. The chicest way to wear a mini is to counter the exposure below the waist with more coverage above. In the winter, a skinny-rib polo neck sweater will give your mini

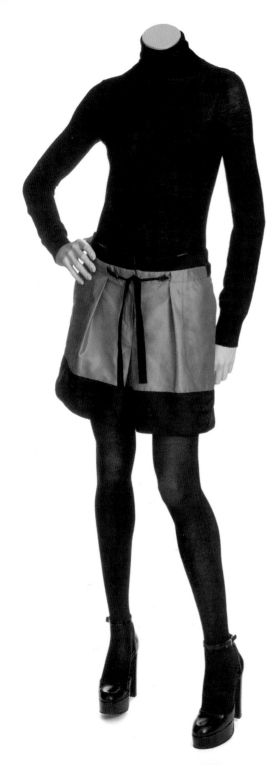

some preppy chic. In the summer, a long-sleeved tunic gives it a bohemian edge.

- It takes serious chutzpah and legs like Bambi to wear a miniskirt and high heels. A softer option is the miniskirt with opaque tights and knee boots.
- A mini that sits on your natural waist can shorten your body. Keep your torso long by positioning the waistband on your hip.
- Flat boots or shoes give your miniskirt some Left Bank spin.

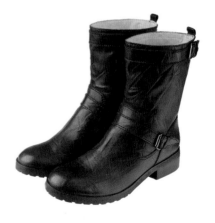

- A leather skirt and leather boots (or an all-suede outfit) is way too much skin. If you live for your leather, then suede boots and a leather skirt (or vice versa) look better.

- If you are wearing a straight skirt and boots, always show some leg between the top of your boots and the hem of your skirt. Full skirts worn with boots don't need the same consideration.

- Baggy-legged boots and any skirt look awful. A boot with a neat leg, and particularly a snug-fitting top, will always look better with your skirt.

## FOR EVENING

An evening skirt is so useful that it's pretty much a wardrobe must-have. By carefully selecting what you wear with it, you can dress it up to the height of formality or down for a bit of languid cocktail glamour.

### 1. Long Evening Skirts

- If you're going long, the most versatile and flattering shape is an A-line. If it sits on the hip bones as opposed to the waist,

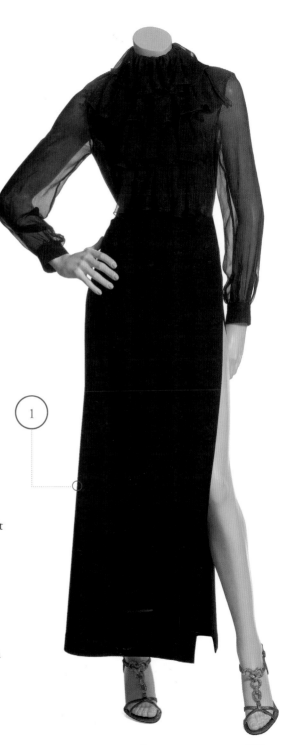

so much the better. It'll give you a little extra length in the torso. Unless you're very tall, avoid long, frilly peasant skirts or anything else with too much volume.

- Avoid flimsy silks and jerseys. A fabric with some substance will smooth your silhouette and give you a clean line from hip to ankle. Wool or rayon crepe will take you anywhere. Velvet is the height of luxury. Duchess satin is sumptuous.

- Success with a long skirt relies on getting the balance right. Lighten the effect of total coverage below the waist with a little exposure on top. It could be something as subtle as a sleeveless shell, V-neck top, or open-necked shirt. If you go for full coverage, you're on the rocky road to frumpsville. The covered-up alternative is a very close-fitting polo neck or round neck, fine-knit sweater, maybe with some extravagant shoes peeping out of that floor-length hem. Close-fitting is the key to sleek, not schlumpy.

2. Short Evening Skirts

- You can go with just about any fabric and shape and still have a very versatile short evening skirt. Use accessories and tops to dress it up or down.

- An extravagantly beaded skirt with a simple T-shirt can do dinner with friends and simply says laid-back glamour. The same item with a silk shell has serious black-tie impact.

- One obvious mistake to avoid is a short evening skirt in a daytime fabric. Matte

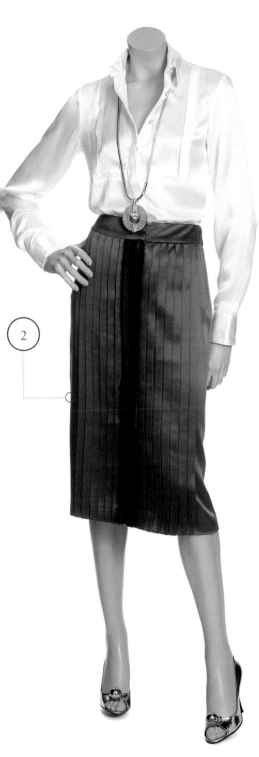

2

wools and jerseys look more comfortable next to a filing cabinet than a Champagne fountain. If you need a skirt that can make the day-to-evening transition, it's better to choose a rayon or silk crepe.

- Bias-cut skirts are feminine and flirtatious and are seriously effective figure smoothers. For maximum figure taming, keep the length on or just below the knee. The longer the line, the slimmer the look.

- Delicate fabrics such as chiffon or lace look their floaty best when laid over a controlling base. If your skirt doesn't have a lining that smoothes over your curves, then invest in a slip that does.

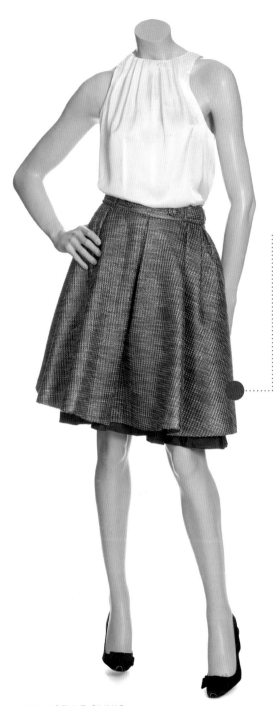

**UNIVERSAL STYLE TRUTH**

A-line skirts look great on everyone.

## HOW TO CHOOSE THE BEST SKIRT FOR YOUR FIGURE

### FLAT BOTTOM

- An A-line will boost your shape best.
- Avoid a straight, tight pencil skirt, which will only emphasize your lack of curves.
- Full skirts are made for women with no bottom. If you're also petite, be sure to emphasise your waist (with a big belt, cummerbund, scarf, or waistband) to keep the volume from swallowing valuable inches in height. Avoid any skirt length below the knee, and wear heels. Even the lowest heel will balance your proportions.
- A slim skirt under a fingertip-length jacket or cardigan will look great. If you keep the jacket and cardigan fairly fluid, the effect is even better.
- The longer the skirt, the more definition your waist and bottom need.

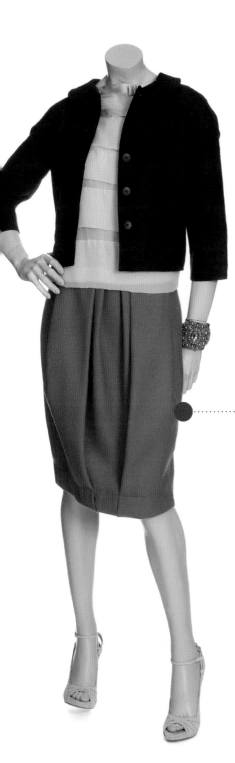

- Oddly, an A-line skirt is a blessing for both curvaceous and boyish figures. For those with larger bottoms, its simple lines work as great hip minimizers.

- A fingertip-length layer (jacket, tunic, cardigan) over a skirt in a fluid fabric worn with high heels is a great proportion-adjuster for women with large hips.

- A well-behaved pencil skirt worn tight can look sexy if it hits a few inches below the knee.

- Pear-shaped women should never cinch their waists. Instead, raise your waistline to make your legs look longer and smooth out the silhouette. Cardigans or shirt jackets buttoned to just above your waist, with the top buttons left undone, will do this.

- For a slim skirt to work for you, it needs to come all the way to the knee, skim (not grip) your hips, and then flare out gently over your bottom.

# 12

## ACCESSORIES

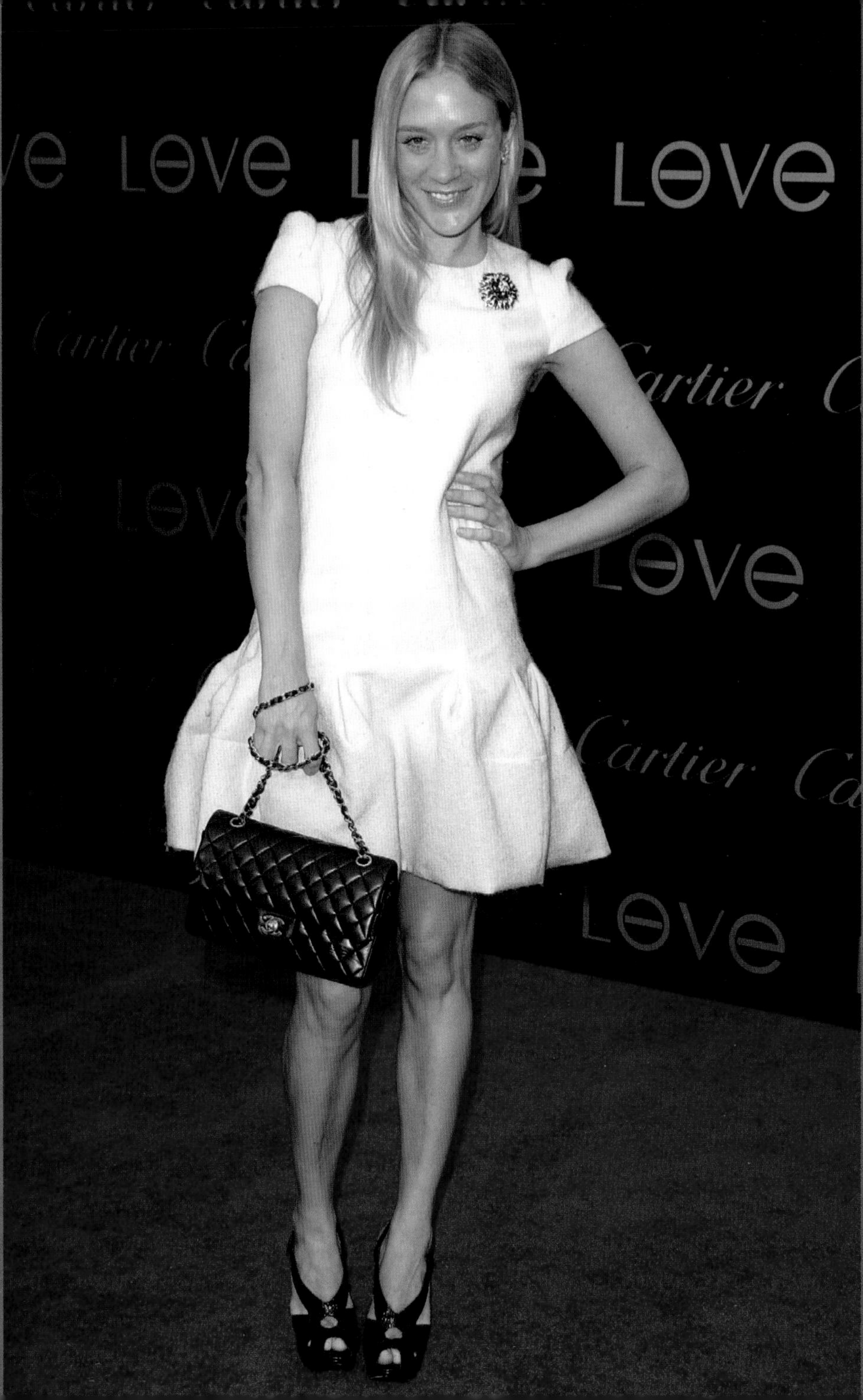
LOVE
Cartier
LOVE
Cartier
LOVE
Cartier
LOVE

**SHOES ARE MORE IMPORTANT** THAN SUITS AND DRESSES. **BUY ONE PAIR OF GOOD SHOES INSTEAD OF THREE PAIR** OF BAD QUALITY.

Marlene Dietrich

GREAT ACCESSORIES make a look memorable. Get the accessories right, and the outfit that goes with them can be as basic as you like. Money is well spent in this department. Sure, you might avoid making a major investment in a shape that will look "last year" before you've even finished paying for it. That aside, even the most extravagant blowout will pay style dividends for decades.

There may be a season or two when prevailing trends force some things to the back of a closet. But you can be sure of this: Your Birkin will be looking fabulous long after those cool pants no longer pass your thighs. No bag will ever make you look fat. No shoes will ever make your butt look big. In my bleakest moments, a shelf full of Manolo Blahniks, Jimmy Choos, and Christian Louboutins have always consoled me more graciously than any cocktail. And, believe me, when your purchasing power is finally spent, a bequest of Blahniks and Birkins will make your daughter, niece, or godchild happier than hard cash.

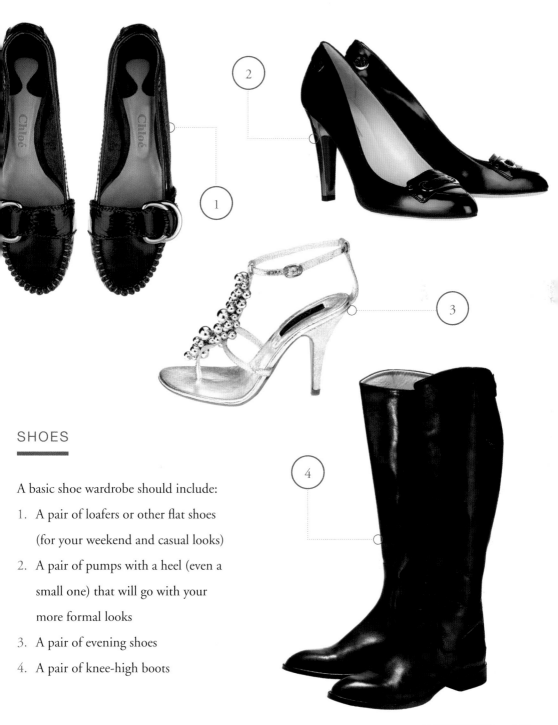

## SHOES

A basic shoe wardrobe should include:

1. A pair of loafers or other flat shoes
   (for your weekend and casual looks)
2. A pair of pumps with a heel (even a
   small one) that will go with your
   more formal looks
3. A pair of evening shoes
4. A pair of knee-high boots

## SHOE SENSE

- Very high heels on short women look out of proportion. Medium height, slender heels are more chic.

- Chunky heels are an essential counter-balance for an outfit with a lot of volume (including wide pants, smock dresses, billowy tunic tops, and thick sweaters).

- Ballet flats are great with cropped slim trousers and miniskirts.

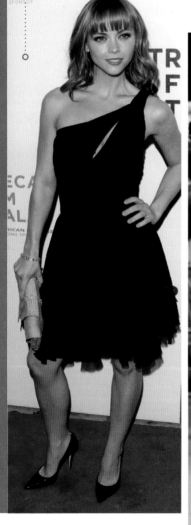
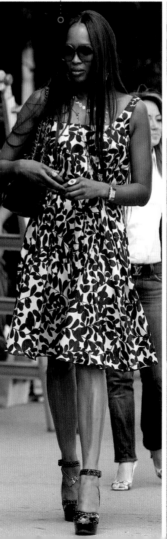
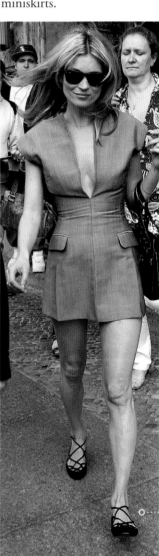

- Roman sandals and leather thongs suit loose looks (caftans, tunic dresses, summer linens).

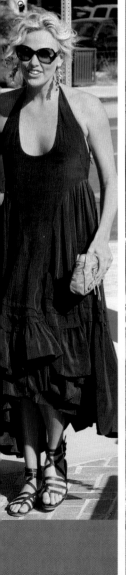

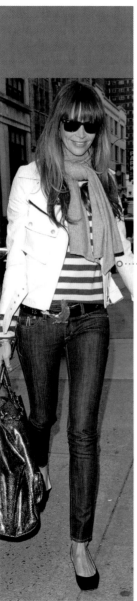

- Loafers and slim-legged trousers or straight-legged jeans are a perfect match. Loafers and a straight skirt work if you are on a preppie nostalgia trip and your legs can take the shortening effect.
- Low-cut pumps flatter thick ankles.
- Wedges slim chunky calves.
- Tall women look great in flats and stunning in heels—as long as they keep their head high and shoulders back.
- Spiky heels look fantastic with light fabrics or slim pencil skirts.

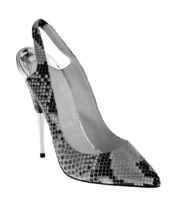

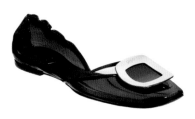

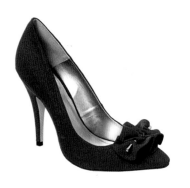

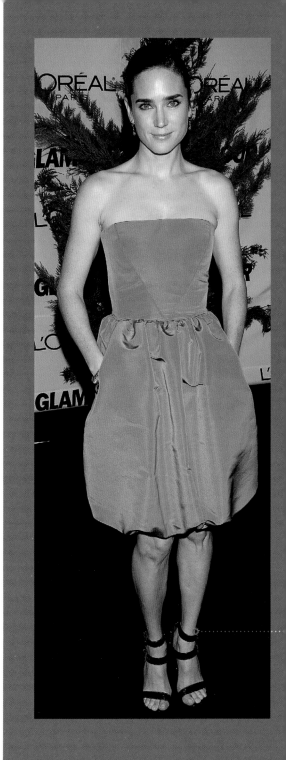

I CAN RUN IN THEM, **I CAN CATCH A TAXI
OR A BUS,** I CAN DO A LOT IN HEELS.
**I CONSIDER MYSELF** A HIGH-HEELED GYMNAST.

Actress Kim Cattrall

- Ankle straps accentuate slim legs, but they also shorten and widen. If in doubt, wear them with longer hemlines (just below the knee if your calves are slender, below the calf or longer if they're not).

- If you are dressing in different tones of the same color, the look is more flattering if the shoes are a darker shade (camel dress with brown shoes or raspberry red dress with burgundy shoes).

- Hosiery with open-toed shoes can work if the hosiery is dense (i.e., opaque or knit). Fishnets work if you can't see the toe seam. And sheer hosiery is okay with closed-toed sling backs. *Never* wear hose and mules.

- Stiletto mules add instant glamour to a summer suit.

- Sculpted heels that look like they are about to mutate or splay at an odd angle look bad with short skirts. Stick to skirts that hit below the knee and trousers.

- Matching bag and shoes are very "mother of the bride."

- Matching accessories were last hot about twenty years ago. If you really must, match your shoes to a piece of your outfit. For example, red shoes will probably work with a print top with red in it. A black dress with red shoes is great. But a black dress with red shoes and a red scarf is not: it's just too contrived.

- High heels lengthen the leg and define the calf muscle—always a good idea.

- Thick-soled shoes with chunky heels are no good on anybody, any time.

## BOOTS

- Tall boots with a heel as high as you can handle are one of the most versatile shapes you can buy. They work under trousers. They look great under slim or full knee-length coats. They look slick with a pencil skirt that hits just on the knee. A bit of leg showing between skirt and boot is a good look as long as you don't have very puffy knees.

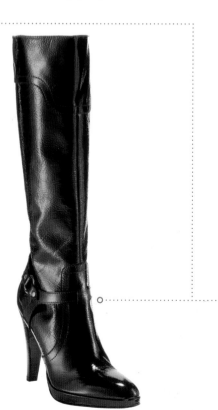

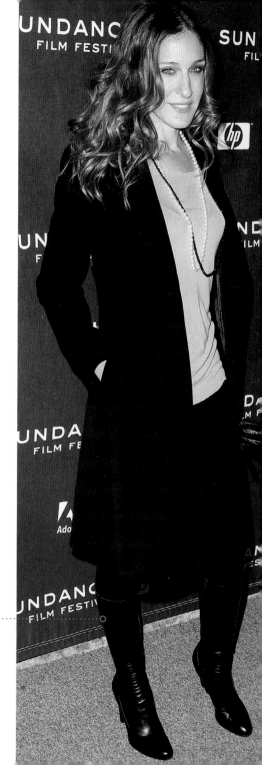

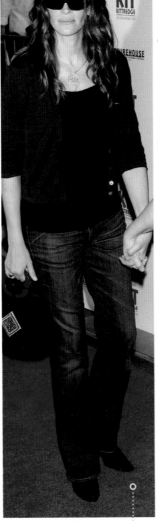

- Flat ankle boots look good with slouchy trousers but generally don't work with skirts unless your legs are fawnlike. Just don't go there.
- Long, slim skirts look good with high-heeled ankle boots.

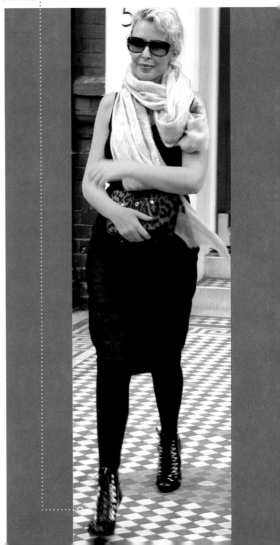

Ankle boots are perfect for under trousers. An ankle boot that sits low, just under the ankle bone, will lengthen your leg if you need the inches. A boot that hits above the ankle will shorten, so be wary.

- Victorian boots have a low heel and a tapered toe and lace up to above the ankle. These look great with cropped trousers (as long as the trouser leg covers the top of the boot), long full skirts, or knee-length A-lines.
- Riding boots are great with full skirts that cover the top of the boot or straight-legged trousers worn over the top. Every so often fashion dictates that they get tucked in. If your legs are on the heavy side, this styling trick will only make them look heavier. Avoid, also, the jodphur/riding boot look unless you are actually out for a hack.

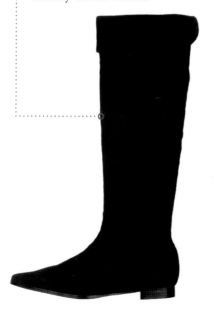

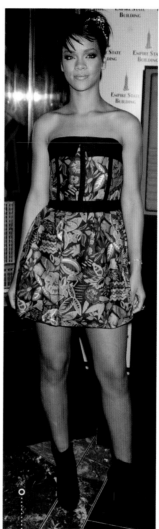

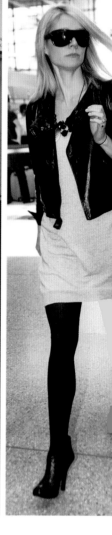

The chunky boot and little skirt is cute on a slim leg. Motorcycle boots work with everything from jeans to lacy dresses and miniskirts.

- Cowboy boots are a classic. Wear them with jeans for authenticity, or go for irony under a sharp suit or romance under a peasant skirt.
- Tall, flat boots can be worn with miniskirts or long flowing skirts, but nothing in between.

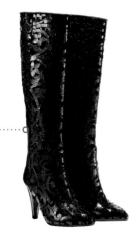

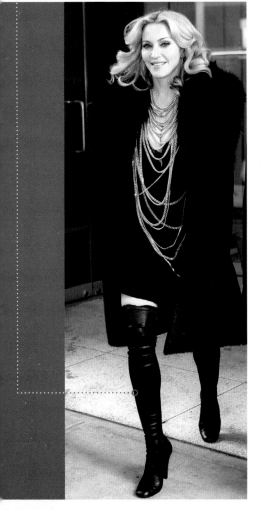

- Evening boots make a powerful impact under long coats or full skirts.

**Get the Perfect Boot Fit**

- The most flattering boot length is the one that hits above the widest part of your calf. The top should be snug, but not digging into your flesh, and the material should have some body, not stiffness.
- A tailored style that skims and therefore streamlines the leg is the best choice for women with big calves. Avoid clingy stretch styles.
- Mid-calf boots are not ideal if you have chunky calves. They hit your leg at its widest point. But if your legs are slim, a mid-calf boot will look great with skirts that hit just above the knee.

## SANDALS

- They're all about the spirit of summer, so make free with style and texture and don't spoil the mood by trying too hard to match colors.

- Money rashly spent on bright-colored shoes is safely invested in bright sandals. They make a neutral outfit special and are ideal for dealing with floral prints.

- When only a neutral will do, try beige or khaki or nude. If that sounds dull, try a neutral reptile. Fake snake and mock croc can look as good as the real thing, and they all make a chic alternative to the simple beige sandal.

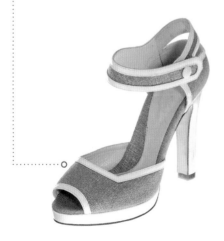

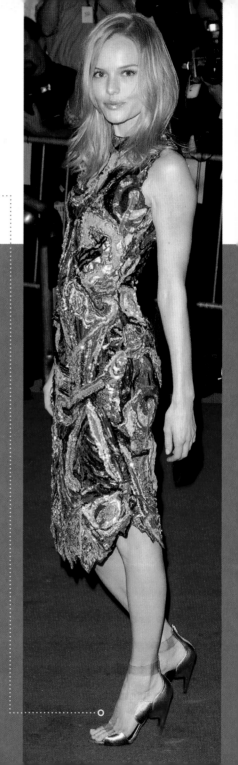

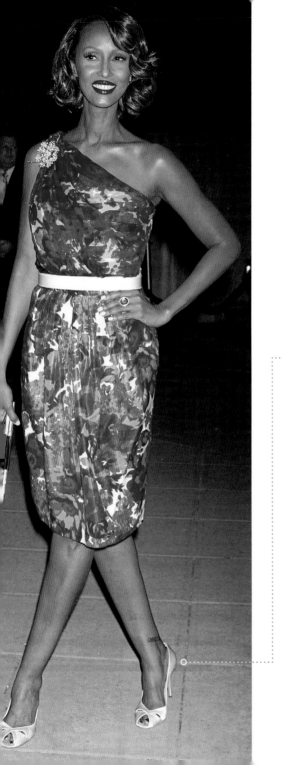

## SHE RAVISHED HIS EYE
## WITH HER SANDALS.

The Bible (on how Judith
distracted Holofernes
before chopping off his head)

- White is not a neutral color in shoes. It's
  a major statement.
- With work clothes, in a conservative
  office, an open, high-heeled sandal
  will still look serious and adequately
  sharp. Flat open sandals in the same
  environment say beach, not boardroom.
- Sandals worn with skirt suits should have
  a heel. If you must wear low or flat heels,
  a closed-toe sandal will look better.
- Foot warning: Never bare your feet or
  toes without first having a pedicure.

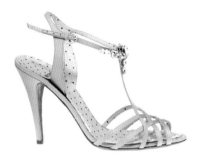

## EVENING SHOES

It's so easy to ruin a great dress with bad shoes. Even if your evening dress comes to the floor and you think you can get away with your old black pumps . . . you can't. Whether or not you can see your feet, someone else surely will. And even if you don't get out much, a great pair of evening shoes is a wardrobe essential. Black evening shoes go with just about anything. Putting them on is enough to signal the shift of your suit or dress from daytime sharp to evening chic. But some shapes are better than others.

- Low-cut shoes and open strappy styles are more slimming than closed high-vamp styles (the vamp is the part that encloses the toe). For fail-safe foot flattery, try a sling-back style or one where the strap angles across the foot from the instep.

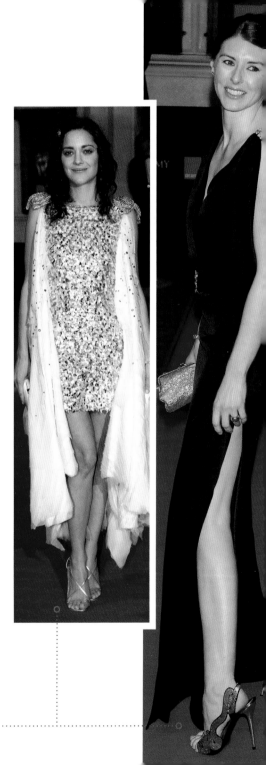

**HIGH-HEELED** THIN-STRAPPED **SANDALS**
HAVE BEEN KNOWN **TO DRIVE SOME MEN**
**TO FRENZIES,** BUT THEY'RE OFTEN MEN
WHO WANT TO TIE YOU UP, SO BE CAREFUL.

Cynthia Heimel, *Sex Tips for Girls*

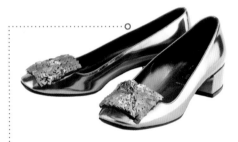

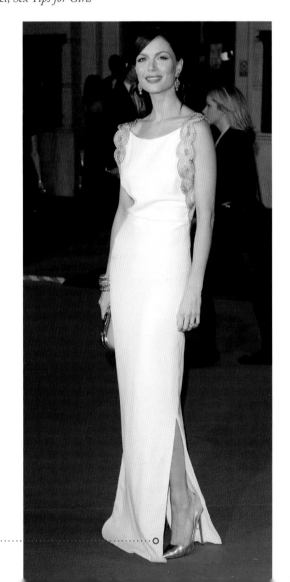

- Flats or a low heel give evening trousers some kicked-back chic. If you're tall, they'll also work with full, ankle-length, ballerina-style skirts.

- The most elegant closed-in style is one that is closed in at the heel and toe but open in between. It's more flattering than a completely closed-in pump, unless you have very wide feet, in which case avoid them (feet spilling over the sides of shoes is never a good look).

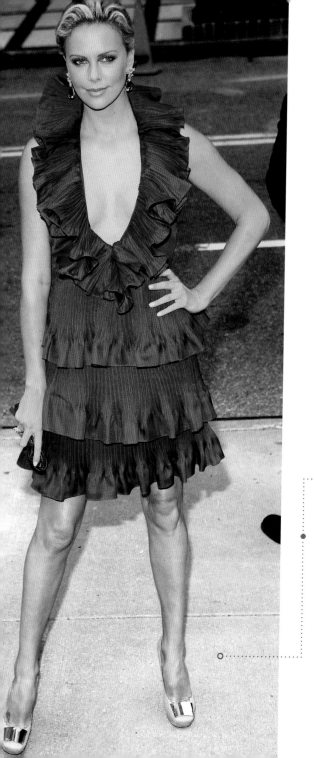

## IF HIGH HEELS
## **WERE SO WONDERFUL,**
## **MEN WOULD BE**
## WEARING THEM.

Sue Grafton, *"I" is for Innocent*

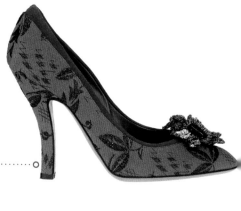

Closed-toed shoes must be cut in a dressy fabric for evening impact. Patent leather, silk, satin, or beaded or decorated fabrics all look better than matte leather or suede, which look as if you forgot you were going out.

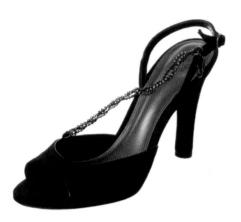

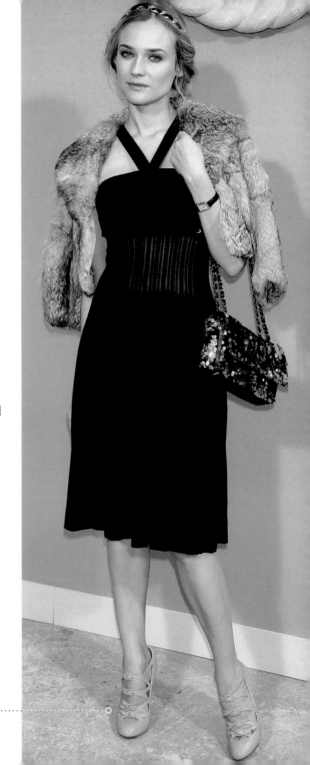

- Evening shoes don't have to be black, silver, or gold. A statement color will add glamour to the most sedate evening classics. If you're nervous, remember: the barer the shoe, the less of an issue its color becomes. The more shine it has (say, satin or patent), the more impact the color has, so if you're going for gloss, make sure you want to make that statement.

- Your feet will look bigger in boldly colorful shoes than dark ones.

## SHOE FIT AND COMFORT

There can't be a woman alive who has never suffered for beautiful shoes. And many go through entire lifetimes believing that being chicly shod is worth the discomfort. A little experience lets you know where the pain is coming from. Most of the list below is not immediately obvious in the shop. Don't say you weren't warned.

- The thicker the heel's tip, the more stable a shoe will feel and the more comfortable it will be to walk/stand around in for hours.

- High heels put more than seven times your body weight on the ball of your foot, so anything that cushions this area will ease the burn. Many companies now add padding under the lining. But, on heels over two inches high, the ball of the foot is under such pressure that you really have to accept that it's beyond anything but token assistance. If you think the shoe is worth it, you simply have to grin and bear it.

- Buy shoes and boots at the end of the day, since your feet expand throughout the day.

- Even if it's a skinny style, the top of your shoes shouldn't pinch your toe. There should always be some wiggle room.

- If you're going for very pointy-toed shoes or boots, you may need to compensate by going up a half or full size.

- The lining should be soft goat, kid, or a high-grade wicking synthetic, not standard synthetics or pigskin, which will cause your foot to sweat and ultimately blister.

- Avoid heat build-up, which also causes discomfort and blistering. The shoe fetishist's best friend is talcum powder. A little sprinkled in your shoe will help keep your feet fresh and dry.

- Get measured regularly. Feet grow as you age. Just because you were a size 9 at twenty doesn't mean you'll still be the same at forty.

- "It'll give a little" is usually a big lie, at least where shoes are concerned. For boots, it's closer to the truth. Because they grip the side and arch of the foot less firmly, the chances of them softening up are slightly better.

- A high-heeled thong will probably cut between your toes.

- Super-thin straps are likely to hurt.

- When trying on shoes or boots, don't walk just on the carpeted area. Try them on a hard surface, too, so you have an idea of how they will feel on the pavement.

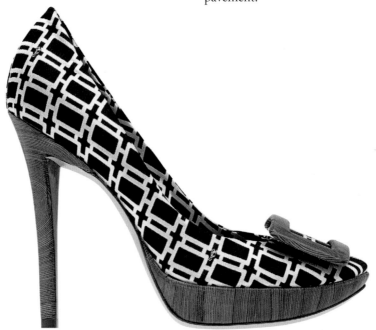

## HANDBAGS

Let's face it: No one bag can do it all for
you. Only a range can cover every angle of
a modern woman's life, from the efficient to
the flirtatious and back again, with a bit of
Bohemian diversion along the way. About
the only rule that matters is to remember
that there are no rules. A bag that matches
an outfit is about the only serious style sin
you can commit in the twenty-first century.
The perfect bag suits your outfit but clashes
just enough: a slouchy bag with a sharp suit
or a psychedelic print bag with a neutral
dress. And don't worry too much about
size. If it works with your look, then a mini
clutch is fine for day, and a tote will work for
the evening.

## WHICH BAG?

What you have in your bag wardrobe will
be dictated largely by your lifestyle: whether
you work in an office or from home, travel,
attend lots of meetings, live in the country
or the city, carry your own stuff or are
responsible for someone else's, too (usually
baby stuff).

If you travel a lot (either long haul or
daily commute by public transport), an
unstructured leather bag in a dark color
will work best. Exterior pockets are good if
you need to keep a phone or tickets handy.
Expandability is helpful as your schlepping
needs vary.

A basic bag wardrobe should include:

1. A smart day bag (to go with suits and
   tailored dresses). Remember that the
   bag that goes with your winter wardrobe
   will look too heavy in the summer, so
   you'll probably need two.

2. A weekend bag (to go with jeans and
   weekend clothes)

3. An evening bag

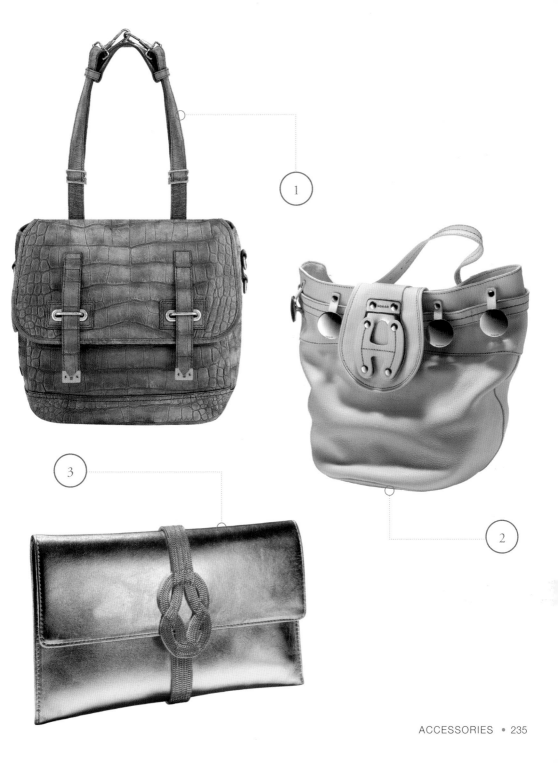

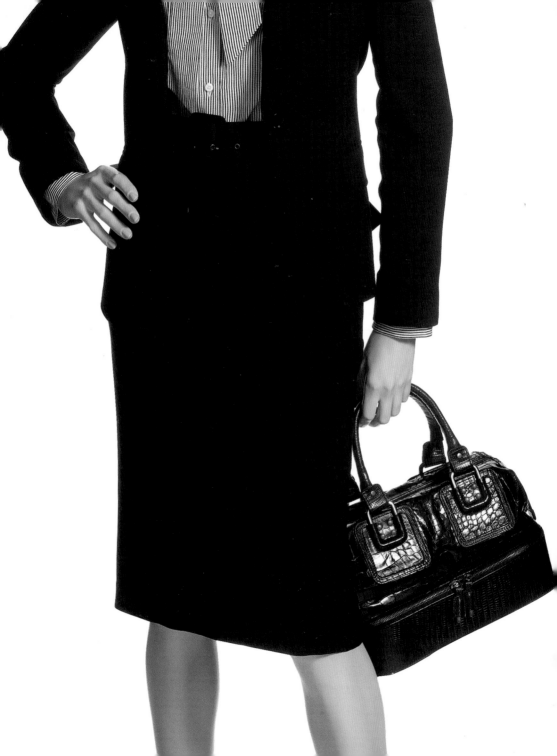

### The Working Bag

This bag carries more responsibility than any other. It's your organizer, your backup, your own personal spin doctor. It presents you to the world at your very best, so don't skimp. A bad bag, like bad shoes, can ruin a positive impression.

- Your bag doesn't have to match your working wardrobe perfectly, but it should put out the same vibe. A backpack might work if your working wardrobe is mostly jeans, but not if you wear suits five days a week.

- The best bag for a drive to work may not be the best one for a commute by public transport. Consider the weight and size and how far you have to walk.

- A great bag should work with your favorite coat(s).

### The Tote

This carryall is the working woman's style ally. It's a fashion workhorse that lets your look be streamlined and clutter free.

- Leather is the best choice by far for durability and glossy good looks. Canvas comes a close second.

- If it feels heavy when empty, imagine what it will feel like full, on a rainy day, on public transport. Think before you buy.

- Make sure it is big enough to carry what you need and that there are enough pockets and dividers.

- Check its shape when full (some bags look really ugly with bulges).

### The Weekend Bag

Nothing looks drearier than a weekday working bag with your weekend clothes. So buy a separate weekend bag. Canvas, slouchy leather, nylon, linen, printed silk, denim, raffia, tweeds, and basket weaves all look great. Live a little!

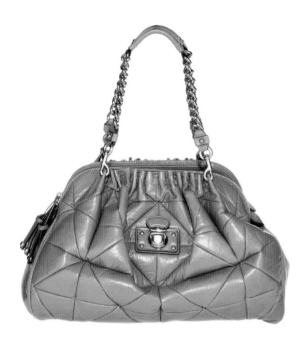

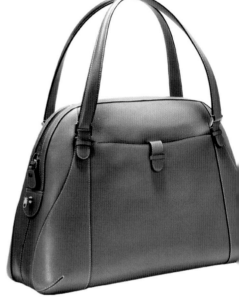

## COLOR

- Black and brown are good neutrals, but not always the best. Khaki or tan will make a better transition from winter to summer.

- A large, bright-colored bag (red, royal blue, or orange) in a classic shape can give a conservative wardrobe serious style impact. But size is key. Anything smaller than a Kelly or Birkin bag looks silly.

- Bright-colored bags are great for diverting attention from your figure, particularly if you wear dark colors.

## STRUCTURE VERSUS SOFTNESS

- Experiment with a shape that is your figure's opposite. If you're round, a streamlined bag gives your look some edge. If you're lean, add curves with a bag that has rounded lines.

- If you want to look boardroom sharp, avoid very unstructured styles. Soft is fine, but smooshy is not.

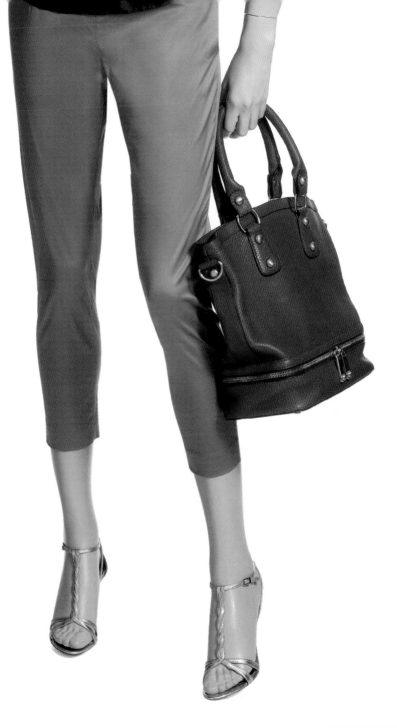

## SIZE

- Your bag should work with your size, not against it. If you're statuesque—either tall, full-figured, or both—a teeny bag will look like a toy and accentuate your size. If you're petite, a really oversize one will look like a magician's prop.

- Small to medium bags look most efficient. A large, overstuffed bag doesn't say hardworking; it says crazed. It also makes you walk like a troll. Stash your stuff in a tote.

## A FEW WORDS ABOUT STRAPS

- If you're busty: Short-strap shoulder bags that snuggle right under your arm, next to your bustline, will do nothing for you. A sleek style that hits you at the waist or a handbag that sits in the crook of your arm is better.

- If you have wide hips: A shoulder bag with a long strap, especially one that bumps right against your hip or is rounded like a bucket, draws attention. A short strap style will flatter and divert the eye upward.

- If you're petite: Short straps work best. Longer versions will drag you down and make you look shorter.

## THE EVENING BAG

- You don't have to invest a fortune in an evening bag. A flea market find is likely to add that ingredient of individuality that upgrades a look from okay to seriously stylish. Beaded, jeweled, or embroidered bags are less likely to show wear and tear and in fact look good even if they are a little distressed.

- Consider what you're wearing, the formality of the occasion, and whether or not you'll need both hands. Don't try to work your way up a receiving line with a drink in one hand and a clutch bag in the other.

- A handbag that dangles from your wrist leaves both hands free. It's ladylike and will fit most of your necessities inside.

- A clutch is the perfect match for a sharp evening look, whether it's a tuxedo or a column or cocktail dress. Take it to sit-down dinners. You can put it on the table and don't have to hold it all night.

- A shoulder bag leaves both hands free but can play havoc with your dress. It doesn't look great with spaghetti straps (too many lines) and it always gets tangled with a shawl. And, no matter how sleek, it always says "cub reporter" in a very formal situation.

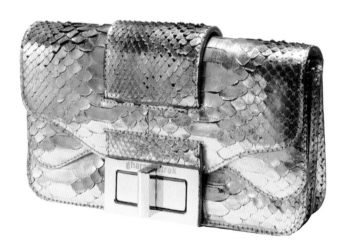

**The Well-Equipped Evening Bag**

You don't need to carry a full makeup kit and a fat wallet. Pare your belongings back to essentials. If you're going out straight from the office, stow what you don't need in a holdall and either leave it in the car or check it at the coatroom. All you really need to have in your bag is:

- Emergency cash (enough to buy a round of drinks or pay for a taxi home)
- A credit and/or debit card
- A portable phone
- Lipstick
- Powder, to blot shine
- A couple of business cards (only if it's a corporate affair)

## ALL-TIME CLASSICS

These bags have all survived the whims of fashion for years. Money spent on any one of them is safely invested.

- Hermès Birkin
- Hermès Kelly
- Gucci hobo bag
- Fendi baguette
- Vuitton tote
- Dior saddle bag
- Chanel 2.55
- Bottega Veneta Minaudier
- Bottega Veneta Cabat

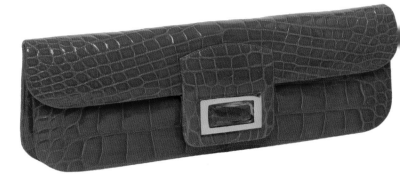

# JEWELRY

The French believe a woman's life story lies in her jewelry box. Every milestone, heartbreak, triumph, and great love, every sentimental and silly moment is represented there. If your jewelry box looks more afternoon soap than big screen epic right now, remember this—every woman deserves a great piece of jewelry. And the days when a girl had to wait to be given it are long gone.

## REAL BASICS

If you've reached the point when the diamanté earrings and plastic watch don't cut it anymore, it's time to think about building a basic fine jewelry wardrobe.

- Pearl stud earrings are a good place to start. They look good with any hairstyle and work as easily with day as eveningwear. They look best either very small or very big. Anything in between is wishy-washy. A real string of pearls that looks good is a major investment. It's priced way beyond what you might expect to invest in a basic fine jewelry wardrobe, so if you like the look, fake it.

- A set of diamond studs are a seriously chic luxury. But anything smaller than 0.5 carats has all the luster of a piece of scrunched up aluminium foil. Diamanté or crystal would look better.

- An elegant watch. Among watch fetishists, the Cartier Tank Francaise (men's or ladies' version, depending on the size of your wrist and hand) and the Rolex Oyster are still firm fashion favorites. But there are so many

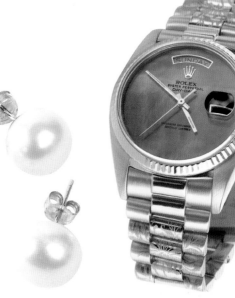

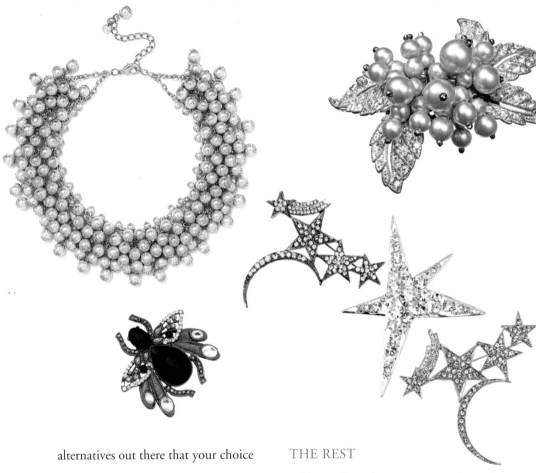

alternatives out there that your choice
is only limited by your budget. Don't
limit your choice to ladies' watches.
A man's watch on a woman's wrist looks
fabulous. Your watch needs to work
equally well with day, evening, and
weekend looks. Whatever you decide,
a gold or stainless steel strap will look
sleek long after a leather strap has given
up the ghost.

## THE REST

Additional jewelry investments depend
on your body and your style. If you have
beautiful hands, maybe you want to make
your statement with rings. If your style is
pretty and feminine, maybe a necklace or
a chain with a diamond drop is what you
need to set off your neckline. If your look
is sporty, then perhaps chunky bracelets
or cuffs are the best way to go. Or maybe

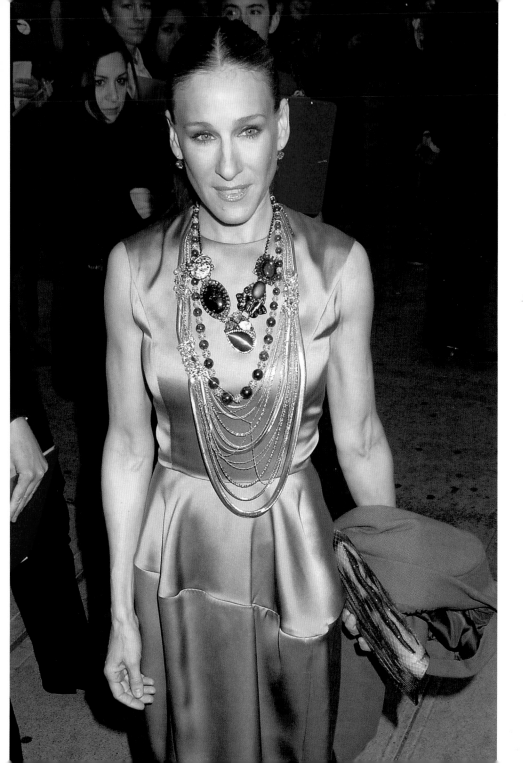

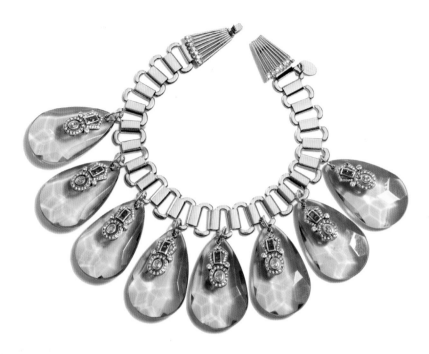

there's a particular designer whose work you love and want to start collecting. Wherever you decide to invest, make sure each item will work throughout your wardrobe. An expensive piece that works with only one outfit is a pointless exercise.

Don't worry about mixing gold, silver, and stainless steel. Matching jewelry has a high frump-factor rating, up there with matching bags and shoes.

## FASHIONABLE FAKES

Thank the fashion gods for costume jewelry. How many tired old outfits have come alive with the timely addition of a rope of colored glass beads or a feathered brooch? The snob value of real over fake is now generations old and not worth a second thought. But if you want to pass off fake as fine jewelry, choose the more delicate settings and keep the stones "real" size.

**JEWELRY** ISN'T MEANT **TO MAKE YOU LOOK RICH,** IT'S MEANT **TO ADORN YOU,** AND THAT'S **NOT THE SAME** THING.

Coco Chanel

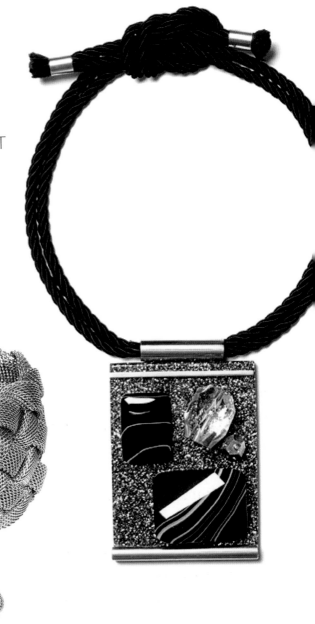

Collect and keep all your flea market finds—you never know when your little black dress will need a boost only that acrylic brooch can give it. But don't expect fashion statements to last longer than the season in which they arrive. Remember the '90s, when all you needed for a big night out was an old nightie and a paste tiara? How we laughed (and still do if there are pictures)! Review your jewelry box once in a while, and stash the gimmicks. The rest has lasting style value.

## HATS

You either are or are not a hat person. But if your only experience is something resembling a flying saucer in papery, pastel-colored straw that you bought in a department store for a wedding, it could be time to reassess.

## HAT FACTS

A hat makes one of the strongest style statements of any accessory. Trouble is, there is precious little middle ground between stunningly good and plain awful. Getting it right comes with experience. But one general rule is that hats are one fashion item that suffer from understatement. The straw hat with the wider brim will always look better than the one that is more conservatively cut. The beret worn at a rakish military tilt wins hands down over the one plonked on your head schoolgirl style. If you're not willing to go for it, then maybe you shouldn't wear a hat at all.

If in doubt, don't shop alone. Take your most honest and stylish friend and that trusty digital camera and have a picture taken in each hat you try. You can make a mirror lie for you, but a camera won't, and having a record of what you tried always helps if you need to think about it. If you're buying a hat for a special occasion, make sure you take the outfit you want to accessorize with you. Here are some ground rules to help you get started:

- Never wear a hat perched on the back of your head. You have to ease it on from the forehead.
- Full figures should go for wide brims.
- Round faces get a lift from the narrow squared-off crown of a fedora or trilby shape.
- Short figures get height from a tall crown. Don't let the brim dip too low or you'll look like the Ant Hill Mob.
- Wide faces suit brimless, off-the-face styles. Berets are great.
- A narrow face needs a rounded, full crown, like a cloche hat.
- Avoid stiff shapes in insipid pastel-colored straw that seem to break out all over department stores like a nasty summer virus. They age everybody. A simple shape in a natural straw is much better.
- Felt is only for winter.

## Hat Proportions

- Statement hat: simple dress
- Cloche hat: calf-length dress
- Veiled hat: sleek dress
- Trilby or fedora: trousers
- Beret: shift dress or slim pants

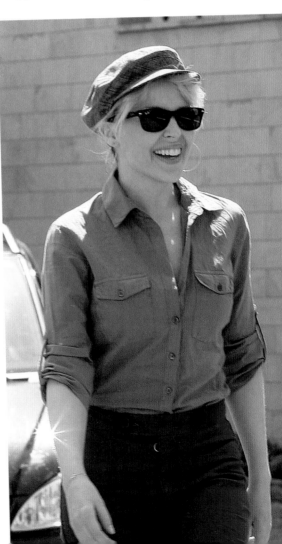

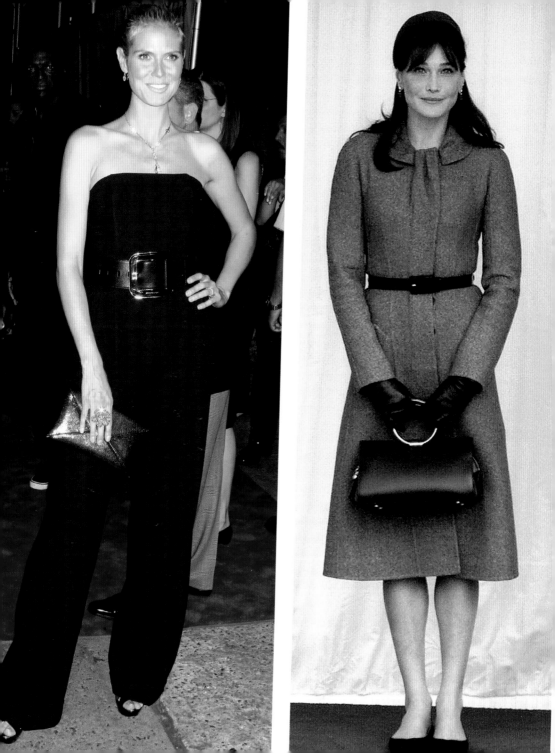

## BELTS

Belts work best when they really bring
something to an outfit. From time to time,
a simple belt can make a strong statement.
A head-to-toe monochromatic look (say a
black or navy suit for the office) can benefit
from the slick line of a leather belt at the
waist. Don't overcinch. Like clothes that are
too small, a too-tight belt will add pounds.

The belts that really earn their wardrobe
space make the difference between an outfit
and a look. A heavy tooled belt slung low
on the hips of a simple silk dress? A pony
skin belt with jeans? An old leather belt with
antique silver buckle cinching a simple shift?
Now we're talking!

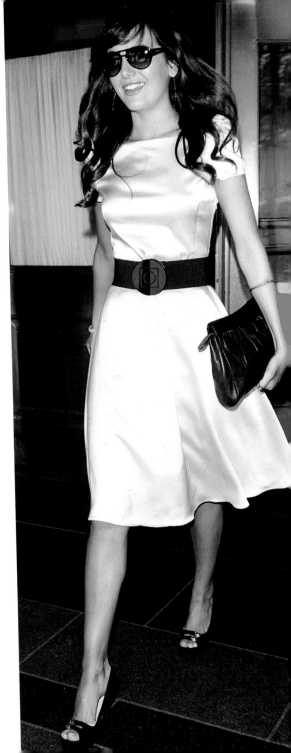

## GLOVES

Gloves are a chic and long-neglected accessory. In the summer, a short pair in pale leather looks fabulous with a shift dress and bare arms. And in the evening they have erotic charm worn long.

Gloves need to be worn with plain and simple lines, and they have to fit your hands and fingers perfectly. The hat-and-glove combo looks wrong unless you're going to church.

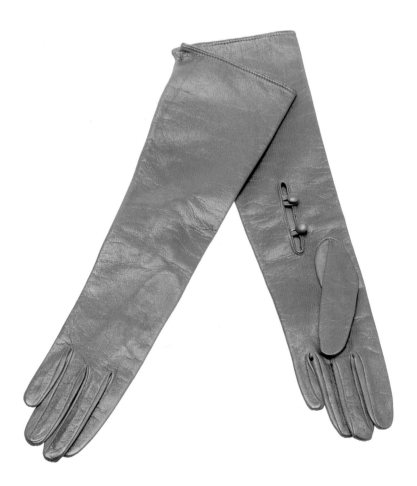

# HOSIERY

If your collection is all about what mom used to wear, you're probably doing your legs no favors. Here are the basic five that should be in every woman's hosiery drawer:

- For bare legs: Nude-colored hose in a matte finish are a key basic (the best brands are Jockey Control Top Sheer Leg, Wolford Logic Pantyhose, Naked 8 Sheer Pantyhose, or Donna Karan Nudes). The matte finish smoothes over uneven skin texture and refines the leg. You can get a sheer effect with good coverage from a thicker knit (look for a higher denier). Shine is for showgirls. You can get away with shiny tights in the evening if they are the only glittery detail in your outfit. But remember, they make all but the best legs look thicker.

- For seductive sheer: Sheer black hose in a matte finish (try Calvin Klein Invisible Comfort or Berkshire Ultra Sheer). Find the brand you like best and buy in multiples so you always have a snag-free pair on hand. Shiny black tights? See above.

- For opaque full coverage: Matte black opaques (try Wolford Synergy or Spanx Tight End tights) are a still a girl's best friend. They slim, smooth, and lengthen the leg. They're almost indestructible (although as soon as they pill, it's time to say goodbye).

- For fishnets: Black micronet fishnets (try Jonathan Aston and Wolford The Twenties) are still chic and sexy after all these years.

## OTHER HOSIERY RULES

- Wear knee-highs under trousers only.
- Sheer stockings work best with similarly delicate shoes. Boots or a chunky shoe will go better with opaque tights.
- Wear stockings that match your shoes, not your skirt. In most cases it looks better, and in all cases it lengthens the leg.

## TEXTURED TIGHTS

Ribbed tights flatter your leg because the vertical lines have a lengthening effect. But almost any other pattern or texture, including big fishnets, will add bulk. Wear them only if you don't mind the extra width. Heavy or exaggerated ribs cancel out their own slimming effect when they wobble over bulges.

## COLORED TIGHTS

Bright colors look great on a runway, an environment that is overlit and inhabited by insect-thin legs. In real life, try burgundy or berry brown instead of scarlet or orange. Try mossy greens and charcoals instead of yellow or royal blue. White tights should never leave the orthopedic ward.

## BARE LEGS

Chic legs can be bare but not look naked. They look best lightly bronzed, but if pale, they should have a baby-smooth and moisturized gleam. Sally Hansen Airbrush Legs or MAC's Face and Body Foundation won't come off on your clothes and work wonders smoothing skin tone. Never go bare-legged in bitter weather unless the time you spend outside is a mere hop from car to a centrally heated venue. Goose-pimply, mottled flesh is never elegant.

## THE LAST WORD

If you worry that your look isn't working perfectly, Coco Chanel's classic advice still applies: before you walk out the door, take one thing off. This usually does the trick. And the excess baggage is more often than not a rogue accessory. When you look in the mirror, pick your point of focus. If it's the silver shoes, let them shine. Don't make them compete with rhinestone hair baubles, a charm bracelet, and half a dozen rings.

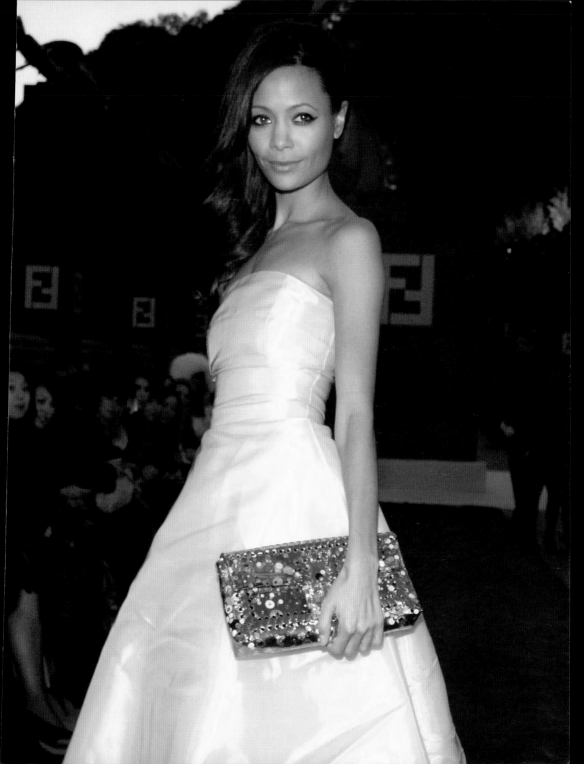

**THE AWARD** FOR PATIENCE AND PERSEVERANCE
in the production of this book must be shared by my editor, Cassie Jones,
and my agent, Elizabeth Kaplan. And for support, encouragement, and stylish
feedback, thanks are due to Evelyn Cohen, Paola Antonelli, Larry Carty, John Reed,
Veronica Herron, Jane Bruton, Johnathan Wilber, Sarah Miller, Sara Rumens,
Stefan Lindemann, Mary and Eliza Bennett, Molly Nyman, Isabella Kullman,
Sue Peart, Charla Lawhon, Dee Nolan, Martha Nelson, Harriet Mays Powell,
Karen Stein, Mary Ellen O'Neill, Amy Vreeland, Paula Szafranski, Susan Kosko,
and Agnieszka Stachowicz. Thanks to Emma Paton and all the good people at
Net-A-Porter for their invaluable help with picture research. And to Alfie and
Finn Munkenbeck, who bravely endured hours of *The Simpsons* while Mommy
was working.

# PHOTOGRAPHY

# CREDITS